Getting to Grips
with
Clinical Governance

Simon Harrison
Colin Pollock
Stephanie Symon

tfm Publishing Limited
Castle Hill Barns
Harley
Nr Shrewsbury
SY5 6LX
UK.

Tel: +44 (0)1952 510061; Fax: +44 (0)1952 510192
E-mail: nikki@tfmpublishing.co.uk; Web site: www.tfmpublishing.co.uk

Design and layout: Nikki Bramhill
First Edition: August 2003

ISBN 1 903378 16 8

Printed by Ebenezer Baylis & Son Ltd., The Trinity Press, London Road, Worcester, WR5 2JH, UK.

Tel: +44 (0)1905 357979; Fax: +44 (0)1905 354919.

Contents

PART IV
Components of clinical governance

APPENDICES

Preface

The history of healthcare in the latter part of the twentieth century is a story of unremitting change. There has been an explosive increase in knowledge, technology and therapeutic options; this has occurred against a background of increasing public expectation coupled with economic restraints on healthcare spending. During this period, the National Health Service (NHS) had to carry the additional burden of repeated organisational change. Much of the political and managerial energy available has been consumed by the need to contain spending while increasing efficiency; quality issues were playing second fiddle. This pattern appeared to change dramatically with the introduction of the concept of clinical governance in the late 1990s.

For many healthcare professionals the introduction of clinical governance was seen as a threat. As new organisations and processes emerged, so did fears of external interference and regulation along with likely erosion of clinical freedom and autonomy. However, others hailed the focus on quality issues as the dawn of a new era and a long-overdue change in emphasis by NHS planners. The passage of time now sees clinical governance established in the vocabulary of everyday medical life but to what extent has the concept changed attitudes, thinking and actions on the shop floor? History will determine whether clinical governance will be seen to be a major turning point in healthcare practices or it will simply form a footnote as being the most popular subject for questions asked during medical interviews in 1998!

This book represents an exploration of clinical governance five years after its introduction and seeks to deliver an understanding of the origins and scope of the concept. The authors have been able to approach the subject from their own, quite different perspectives within the NHS. Hospital practice, at both senior and junior level, general practice and public health medicine are represented. The aim has been to include a critical and, at times, opinionated analysis of how doctors, nurses, health service managers and co-workers can adapt to and develop with this new, quality-orientated agenda. It is our belief that there is a serious risk that clinical governance may fall into disrepute as being a bureaucratic nuisance inflicted on over-stretched workers in a top-down manner. The alternative is for clinical governance to be used in a constructive way as the counterbalance that protects the quality of patient care from the pressures of cost-containment and the calls to process patients more rapidly and in ever-greater numbers. We hope that this book will go some way to helping its readers develop the clinical governance concept into a practically-based way of thinking about and delivering care to their patients.

One difficulty faced by the well-intentioned individual who wishes to keep abreast of developments in the quality agenda is that of information overload. Furthermore, this is a rapidly changing environment so that the various agendas are continuing to develop month by month. In order to help sort the wheat from the chaff in the volumes of literature that are being produced we have provided suggestions for further reading. We hope that these additional resources will help the reader to flesh out the subject.

Acknowledgements

We are very grateful to Nikki Bramhill, our editor, for her direction and enthusiasm throughout this project, to Phil Ayres and Ann Christian for comments on early drafts and to Gillian Richardson for her invaluable input on audit. Our appreciation also goes to colleagues in the Department of Urology at Pinderfields Hospital for their ongoing support. Finally, we are indebted to our families, without whose patience and encouragement this book would not have been written.

Authors

Mr Simon Harrison was appointed in 1992 as Consultant Urologist with a special interest in Spinal Injury to Pinderfields Hospital, Wakefield. He has been involved in extensive developments within the hospital's urological and spinal injury services and has maintained an active role in both teaching and research. Further insights into the workings of the Health Service were gained from serving as chairman of the Trust's Senior Medical Staff Committee. He is married with two children.

Dr Colin Pollock is Deputy Regional Director of Public Health in the Yorkshire & Humber Region. He began his professional career in general practice in Otley, West Yorkshire, before moving to public health medicine in 1989. He has worked as Director of Public Health for Wakefield Health Authority and Eastern Wakefield Primary Care Trust. He is married with two children.

Miss Stephanie Symons is a Urology Specialist Registrar, training in London. She undertook her basic surgical training in Manchester, Leicester and Reading before working as a research registrar in Pinderfields General Hospital, Wakefield. She lives with her partner in north-west London.

PART I

The origins of quality in the NHS

Any attempt to understand and engage with the clinical governance concept is doomed to failure unless one has some appreciation for its historical context. The chapters in Part I summarise the development of the NHS and examine how issues of healthcare quality have been dealt with over time. Clinical governance has not been discovered, like some strange new species; it has developed in response to historical, social and professional pressures. Any sense of novelty owes more to the choice of name than to the underlying components themselves, although the impact of this new focus on quality has been dramatic.

Chapter 1

Modern expectations of healthcare

Changed, changed utterly: a terrible beauty is born.
WB Yeats

If clinical governance is about providing quality patient care, then what is new about that? Since its launch in 1948 the National Health Service (NHS) has been committed to providing modern healthcare to all that cross its threshold. And over the past 50 years it has done a remarkable job. It has banished many of the fears that had accompanied illness and, as the politicians repeatedly remind us, NHS staff treat one million people every day [1]. Doing the best for the patient has long been the mantra of the healthcare professional and all will recount tales of personal sacrifice which have arisen from a desire to fulfil this pledge.

But the past 50 years have also seen enormous change, both within healthcare and society. And in the face of change no organisation, however great or dedicated, can afford to stand still. The traditional 'quality service' provided by the NHS has now been brought into question and 'quality' in healthcare has begun to be redefined. The NHS must be prepared to change and to focus on the things that really matter to the public it serves.

The challenges faced by health providers are now greater than ever. Internationally medicine continues to advance at an enormous pace. Any modern health service must keep up-to-date with this rapid change. Further, it must rise to the challenge of serving a more informed and demanding public.

Bearing witness to the last 20 years of health service policy has made the 21st century public more likely than ever to question the ability of the

NHS to serve its cause. The internal market, which highlighted regional disparities in provision of care, unsurprisingly angered those unable to access services available in neighbouring areas. Additionally, well-publicised service inefficiencies have not matched up to the public expectation of a service in line with the rapid, modern world. And a decade marred by several high profile medical disasters has further undermined public confidence in health.

With the arrival of the New Labour government in 1997, the NHS was presented with a fait accompli: the modernisation programme. The acceptance that the NHS had been subjected to chronic under funding was accompanied by a political belief that lack of resources was not the only NHS ailment; there was also a need to introduce reform to the systems, practices and culture of the health service. Variations in health practice which have become commonplace are no longer viewed as being acceptable and consistency in the quality of healthcare is demanded.

The government's modernisation objective is to ensure fair access to high quality care for all patients wherever they are treated within the NHS. Patients should now be able to benefit from national standards in health, while retaining the privilege of individualised care. The modernisation programme has made standardisation, provision and monitoring of quality patient care a statutory duty for health providers. Thus, the quality of patient care, which for so long has been implied, must now be assured. Clinical governance is the vehicle by which this is to be achieved and there is definitely something new about that.

However, this quality initiative did not arrive overnight as the brainchild of a new government. It is the culmination of changes that have occurred over more than 50 years. To understand further the roots of this development it is useful to look briefly at the history of the NHS and the evolution of modern medical practice, as well as the changing demands of patients and society as a whole.

References

1 The New NHS, Modern, Dependable. Secretary of State for Health. The Stationery Office, London, December 1997.

Further reading

• Secretary of State for Health. The NHS plan. A plan for investment. A plan for reform. The Stationery Office, London, 2000. www.nhs.uk/nhsplan.

• Smith R. All changed, changed utterly. *BMJ* 1998; 316: 1917-1918.

• Berwick DM, Enthoven A, Bunker JP. Quality management in the NHS: the doctor's role - I. *BMJ* 1992; 304: 235-9.

• Berwick DM, Enthoven A, Bunker JP. Quality management in the NHS: the doctor's role - II. *BMJ* 1992; 304: 304-8.

• Berwick DM. Continuous improvement as an ideal in healthcare. *N Engl J Med* 1989; 320: 53-56.

• Scally G, Donaldson LJ. Clinical governance and the drive for quality improvement in the new NHS in England. *BMJ* 1998; 317: 61-65.

Chapter 2

Creating a national service for health

Never mind the quality, feel the width.
Anon

The creation of the NHS in 1948 was to erase the disparity in healthcare that had gone before it. A comprehensive, state-run healthcare system was one inevitable conclusion of the enormous social and political reform that had occurred during the previous century. Table 1 highlights some of the key moments in the history of healthcare which led towards the creation of the NHS and followed its inception.

The origins of welfare

The beginnings of the welfare state had been in the Poor Law reforms of the mid-19th century. The speed of evolution then increased dramatically into the early 20th century. There were two main drivers for change. Firstly, the poor health amongst military volunteers during the Boer War (1899-1902) led to an increasing fear of national degeneration. National well-being and the security and glory of the British Empire were of major concern [1]. Secondly, the more educated and liberal attitudes of powerful social philanthropists had highlighted the injustice and waste of individual poverty. In response, society increasingly viewed the poor as deserving rather than as morally corrupt. Shock reports by Booth [2], Rowntree [3] and various Royal Commissions on the state of the nation's health, added further fuel to the social reform fire.

Thus, the early 20th century was a period of dramatic social reform, with increased support for children, widows, the elderly and the unemployed. But despite this enormous tide of change, the poorly funded

Table 1. Key moments in healthcare.

Royal College of Physicians established	1518
Royal College of Surgeons established	1800
Poor Law and Public Health Acts	1834/75
General Medical Council formed	1858
School Medical Service began	1907
GP panels established in the National Insurance Act	1911
World War I	1914/18
General Nursing Council established	1919
'A General Medical Service for the Nation' published by BMA	1928
World War II	1939/45
Beveridge report on the 'five giants' of need published	1942
NHS established	1948
Enoch Powell's Ten Year Hospital Plan	1962
Family Doctors Charter (new national contract for GPs)	1966
NHS re-organisation	1974
- NHS takes over community health services from local authorities	
- Community Health Councils established	
NHS re-organisation	1983
- Introduction of general managers to NHS	
NHS re-organisation	1991
- Introduction of NHS Trusts, GP fundholding, the purchaser-provider split and formal clinical audit for doctors	
Bristol Paediatric Heart Surgery Inquiry	1996
Harold Shipman arrested	1997
Medical (Professional Performance) Act	1997
NHS re-organisation	1997
- 'End of the internal market', GP fundholding abolished, Primary Care Trusts established	
- Clinical governance launched	
National Institute for Clinical Excellence and Commission for Health Improvement established	1999
National Clinical Assessment Authority established	2001
Alder Hey Inquiry Report published	2001
National Patient Safety Agency established	2001
Modernisation Agency established	2001

and disparate health services became increasingly unable to combat the poverty and disease which still remained. By 1939, following World War One and the depression of the inter-war years, the state of the hospitals and General Practitioner (GP) services was desperate.

Health services prior to the Second World War

Most GP practices at this time were single-handed and deputising services were non-existent. GPs worked for long hours and in isolation. Their livelihood relied on seeing patients who were able to pay them and this added to the erratic nature of care. Within the hospital sector, the service available was no more uniform. Hospitals, which relied on either voluntary contributions or central government payments through patient means testing, were all sorely under-funded and provided markedly differing levels of care.

Despite increased social support, a significant section of the population remained poor. Access to the healthcare system was essentially based on means so that many kept their distance from doctors through an unwillingness or inability to pay. Prior to the launch of the NHS, healthcare was at best haphazard and at worst non-existent.

A vision of a national health service

When war broke out in 1939, the structure of welfare and health provision changed. The new coalition government had to bring in urgent measures to ensure that the country kept running despite the war. This meant that the pre-war market pressures were overridden in order to ensure that basic human needs were being met. The systems, which had been based on the concept of means, were now replaced with a system based on universality and need. Early in the war, family welfare was developed, with free milk, free immunisation and subsidised school meals. The Emergency Medical Service was created to link the voluntary and state hospitals in order to cope with war casualties in a more integrated and planned way. This was the first time that anything like a uniform health service had existed. By the end of six years of war, the enormous benefits of state run organisations were well recognised by those in power.

By 1945, the establishment of a national health service was inevitable. Now that people had seen that it was possible, there was no going back to the pre-war ad-hoc nature of hospital provision. Beveridge's 1942 social security report [4] had denounced the 'five giants' of 'Disease, Squalor, Ignorance, Idleness and Want'. This in turn had led to a White Paper in 1944 [5] which stated: "Everybody, irrespective of means, age, sex or occupation shall have equal opportunity to benefit from the best and most up-to-date medical and allied services available". The scene was set for the new peacetime government to push through a raft of welfare legislation whose origins lay a century earlier, but which war had made possible.

Quality or quantity?

But what about quality in healthcare? Throughout this entire period of social reform, the quality of care provided had not been questioned. It was always a case of 'the more the better' or 'never mind the quality, feel the width'. Quality was implicitly guaranteed because of the unrivalled status of the medical profession.

This was poignantly illustrated in the establishment of the NHS, where the primary focus was again on provision of care. In 1948 Bevan launched the NHS and in a message to doctors he stated:

"My job is to give you all the facilities, resources, apparatus and help I can, and then leave you alone as professional men and women to use your skill and judgement without hindrance" [6].

In post-war Britain, which had relied so heavily on the expertise of the medical and nursing professions during the years of combat, the assumption of quality within care went unchallenged. But history has shown that such professional freedom does not last and issues of quality control have since come increasingly to the fore.

The NHS: a perfect solution?

In the years following 1948, the stark realities of the financial bottomless pit which is healthcare, began to be recognised. This led to the rapid reintroduction of health charges, initially for prescriptions and dental work. And as local government struggled to manage the financial burden of the NHS, the national uniformity of care was inevitably put under stress.

At the same time, a post-war generation grew up with the expectation of free and available healthcare. Within this new society, information technology allowed the public to witness the enormous progress made in medicine, as well as many notable medical failures.

So, just as the social and political reforms of the first half of the century had highlighted the need for a national health service, the ensuing social and technological advance made clear the need for further reform within health.

References

1   Royle E. *Poverty and Welfare in: Modern Britain. A Social History 1750-1985*. Edward Arnold (Ed), 1989: 157-226.

2   Booth C. *Life and Labour of the People of London*. Macmillan, London, 1903.

3   Rowntree S. *Poverty: A Study in Town Life*. Macmillan, London,1901.

4   Beveridge Report. Social Insurance and Allied Services. Command Paper 6404. HMSO, London, 1942.

5   A National Health Service. Command Paper 6502. HMSO, London,1944.

6   Bevan Aneurin. A message to the medical profession from the Minister of Health. *The Lancet* 1948; 2: 24.

Further reading

•   The Bristol Royal Infirmary Inquiry. Annex A, chapter 2. A Historical Background to the NHS. www.bristol-inquiry.org.uk/final_report.

•   Rivett G. *From Cradle to Grave: Fifty Years of the NHS*. Kings Fund, London, 1998.

•   NHS 50th Anniversary Resource Pack. Address for correspondence: Communications Unit. NHS Executive, Quarry House, Quarry Hill, Leeds LS2 7UE.

Chapter 3

Changing professional practice and attitudes

God and the doctor we alike adore
But only when in danger, not before;
The danger o'er, both are alike requited,
God is forgotten, and the Doctor slighted.
John Owen

In 1948 Aneurin Bevan handed the reins of the newly created NHS to the doctors and nurses who would run it. Few could have envisaged how dramatically their professional lives would change over the years that followed. Sub-specialisation, controlled hours through working time directives and increasing litigation have all played their part in the evolution of the modern service. The following paragraphs illustrate some of the ways in which professional life has altered and the stresses on service quality which have emerged as a result.

The loss of the generalist

It was only with the passing of the Medical Act of 1886 that it became a requirement for doctors to be qualified in medicine, surgery and midwifery. The joining of these historically individual trades gave birth to the generalist, most notably in the form of the general practitioner. But this overarching method of medical practice has lasted less than a century.

Although most General Practitioners (GPs) have continued to administer medical, surgical and obstetric care to patients in the community, the extent of the service provided has becoming increasingly narrow. The modern primary healthcare centre is a far cry from the days when all GPs regularly performed surgery and delivered children at home.

In secondary care also, individual doctors have become increasingly limited in the scope of care that they provide. And now, in the 21st century, sub-specialisation is the norm.

Increasing specialisation has been a natural response to rapid changes both within and outside medicine. Advances in medical knowledge, technology and techniques have made it increasingly difficult for doctors to remain competently on top of their field. Without knowledge, doctors lose the status that comes with professional expertise. Furthermore, faced with an increasingly educated and informed public, a convincing position as expert has become harder to retain. Thus, the only way for doctors to maintain the ability to provide a quality specialist service to patients has been to limit their field of practice.

The benefits of specialisation are obvious, but the narrowing of professional practice does carry some risks. For example, it is increasingly difficult to staff emergency services with practitioners who are trained and up-to-date in all the areas of medicine that they may need to cover; the patient with a bleeding ulcer may well find themselves under the care of a doctor whose interests and skills lie in the management of diabetes rather than gastroenterology.

A limited working life

But it is not only in their subject that modern doctors have become limited. The working week has also been significantly reduced. Only 10 years ago junior doctors were still regularly working more than twice the hours that are now deemed acceptable. Within a working environment that left very little space for outside activity, medicine remained a vocation and doctors had no choice but to be committed to their work first and foremost. However, the militancy of modern juniors together with United Kingdom entry into the European Union has secured better pay and conditions of service for all doctors [1]. This is undoubtedly a step forward, but has not come without drawbacks.

The reduced working day of the junior doctors has had several knock-on effects in terms of quality service provision. One of the most prominent complaints to have arisen from the working time directive is the loss of continuity in care. Historically, a single junior had been responsible for a patient throughout the admission process and their subsequent hospital stay. In comparison, current shift patterns can lead to an individual patient being looked after by three or four junior doctors in turn. The introduction of these new working patterns has not always been accompanied by a review of the system to which they have been applied. This has resulted in concerns over patient safety in the potentially chaotic clinical environment; such a rapid turnover of staff brings enormous potential for errors in communication and clinical care.

A further anxiety which has arisen as a result of the reduction in working hours relates to the impact of such changes on training. Shorter and less varied training may have eroded the ability of doctors to gain the extensive hands-on experience that has previously been heavily relied upon. Reform of medical training has been implemented but its effectiveness in countering this threat is far from being established. There are real concerns that some newly appointed consultants will be expected to demonstrate skills and a clinical maturity that their training has simply not provided; the resulting clinical fallout would precede further rounds of litigation and consultant suspensions.

Defensive practice

Thus, sub-specialisation and limited working hours have led, of necessity, to new methods of medical practice. In order to maintain expert status, health professionals are becoming increasingly less likely to take responsibility for any aspect of patient care that is outside what they see as their remit. But more than anything, it has been the fear of public recrimination, which has now taken this change in medical practice to a new level. The incessant rise in the frequency of complaints and litigation has been one of the most significant modern developments that the health service has had to face.

The increased legal challenges over the past 20 years have led to a reactive increase in defensive practice. Where in the past, it was rare to experience any form of litigation within a career, it is now so commonplace as to be regarded as normal. In a working environment where adverse events are so often perceived as avoidable clinical errors, the behaviour of clinicians is driven, not only by positive motivations, but also by a reflex desire to save their own professional skins.

The financial, personal and professional cost of defensive practice is inevitably high. Patients will find themselves submitted to increasing numbers of expensive and invasive investigations, which may enhance neither the accuracy of diagnosis nor the outcome of treatment. They will also find themselves under the care of an increasingly confusing array of professional teams. For health professionals, training now inevitably covers issues of complaints and litigation. Consequently, high-risk specialties that were once so desirable may now find themselves out of favour as junior doctors increasingly seek out training in less traumatic areas of clinical practice.

21st century healthcare

And so, 50 years following its creation, the NHS relies upon a breed of health professional very different from those who first directed its path. Gone are the days of the confident, unchallenged generalists, dedicated to the health service first and foremost. In their place are specialists, now keenly aware of their more tenuous relationship with the modern public and defensive in response.

But with the announcement of clinical governance, NHS staff have been given the opportunity to tackle many of their service concerns as well as their relationship with the public. The quality and efficiency issues raised internally by sub-specialisation, reduced hours and defensive approaches to practice can now be given a formal airing in the light of modernisation.

References

1   Guidance on Working Patterns for Junior Doctors. A document produced jointly by the Department of Health, the National Assembly for Wales, the NHS Confederation & the British Medical Association. Department of Health, London, November 2002. Available at www.doh.gov.uk/workingtime.

Further reading

- Friedson E. The Formal Characteristics of a Profession. In: *Profession of Medicine. A study of the sociology of applied knowledge.* Chicago, III. University of Chicago Press, 1988: 71-84.
- Irvine DH. The Performance of Doctors. Professionalism and self regulation in a changing world. *BMJ* 1997; 314: 1540-2.
- Berwick DM, Enthoven A, Bunker JP. Quality management in the NHS: the doctor's role - I. *BMJ* 1992; 304: 235-9.
- Berwick DM, Enthoven A, Bunker JP. Quality management in the NHS: the doctor's role - II. *BMJ* 1992; 304: 304-8.
- Learning from Bristol: report of the public inquiry into children's heart surgery at the Bristol Royal Infirmary 1984-1995. The Stationery Office, Norwich, 2001.
- Supporting doctors, protecting patients. A consultation paper on preventing, recognising, and dealing with poor clinical performance of doctors in England. Department of Health, London, 1999 (www.doh.gov.uk/cmoconsult1.htm).

Chapter 4

Changing public demands

Come gather 'round people wherever you roam
And admit that the waters around you have grown
And accept it that soon you'll be drenched to the bone.
If your time to you is worth savin', then you better start swimmin'
Or you'll sink like a stone, for the times they are a-changin'.
Bob Dylan

There is a stark contrast between the patient whose approach is encapsulated by "whatever you think is best doctor" and the individual who arrives in clinic clutching a sheaf of papers detailing the latest international thinking on their condition. This new breed of NHS patient is part of a growing minority which has taken significant getting used to. The demands placed on the service from informed and questioning patients are undoubtedly higher than those placed by the traditional, standard NHS patient.

Of course, this is just one manifestation of the trend towards a modern, educated and less accepting public, a trend that has been growing over many years. What has driven this development and how has it impacted on the need for modernisation in health?

Familiarity breeds contempt

The arrival of the NHS followed six years of international war and decades of economic hardship for the majority of the British population. Its arrival brought hope and a new prosperity to those who had gone without for so long. Overnight the people of Britain were given a step up to health. Suddenly free glasses, hearing aids, prescriptions and dental care were available; all of these made enormous changes to the lives of people who had previously had low expectations of healthcare and had accepted significant suffering as a matter of course.

But time moves on and over a 50-year period, the proportion of the population that remembers life without a national health service is ever shrinking. This experience extends further. Society is now used to an extensive welfare system which extends, to a greater or lesser degree, from birth to old age. The generations brought up with the expectation of free healthcare now take this privilege for granted and, as the saying goes, familiarity breeds contempt.

Society in general no longer views a free health service, or indeed unemployment benefit, child benefit or the state pension, as a privilege - these are now expected as a right. This powerful change in attitude towards the welfare system has had a tremendous knock-on effect. The pressure on public services grows inexorably as the public develops ever-greater expectations of their effectiveness and becomes reliant on their provision. And any service that is presumed to be a right is ripe for public criticism. Both pressure and criticism grow together as public services strain under the weight of public demand.

Knowledge equals power

But it is not familiarity with the health service and our increasing dependence upon it which leads to the patient arriving in clinic with a weighty Internet brief. The education provided over the past 50 years has changed the face of society forever. The Education Act of 1944 laid the foundation and set out the principle of education for all, regardless of class. The result of educational reform has been an increasingly informed and aware population.

Health education has been fed to the nation in both formal and informal ways. Within schools, physical, sexual and mental health are all now represented in the curriculum. Outside the formal education system, the media continuously feeds us with information about health matters. Indeed, there is a frenzied interest in healthcare stories. There is media encouragement to take part in national screening programmes along with documentaries that detail the life of our hospitals and a host of agony aunts to answer the nation's health questions.

This access to individual knowledge has empowered modern patients. Those using the health service now find themselves in a position of some understanding of the issues that involve them. From this position patients are better able both to question and to criticise the service which is being delivered. They are also more likely to demand an individualised service or one that they have seen advertised elsewhere.

Globalisation

International health news and the Internet have more recently taken health education to an even higher level. Not only do the public have an increased awareness of their own health and the usual practices within the United Kingdom (UK), but also there is now extensive knowledge about what is available on a global scale. Many of the health technologies which patients are seeing advertised, occur at the boundaries of medical possibility, in some of the most well-funded and innovative centres on the planet. However, this does not inhibit the public from believing that such treatments are available to them or that they should be.

This mass marketing of medical ideas also has a profound effect on the public's belief in the power of medicine to treat any ill. The acceptance of and increasing reliance upon chemical compounds to cure illness is a good example of this. It also typifies the way that scientific research and practice in society has developed over the last 300 years. The scientific thinking that has dominated the 20th century has led us to expect a cure for all diseases. There is an expectation that observation and measurement will lead to an explanation of cause and effect. By looking long and hard enough we expect to always find an answer. Within medicine, this search has continued increasingly at molecular and sub-molecular levels. Patients have not been immune from such thinking and now also expect modern science and medicine to hold the answers. Every disease and illness should have its explanation, and cure.

Consumerism

Within the UK there has been a further profound influence on the public's belief that an efficient, effective and high quality service is to be expected at every health centre within the UK: the Patient's Charter [1]. With its launch by John Major at the beginning of his term of office, the public suddenly had black and white evidence of the service that they should expect. Patients could now quote acceptable waiting times for first appointments and treatment regimes. In addition they were advised exactly what standard of care they could expect to receive during a hospital admission, from the communication skills of the staff to the nutritional value of the meals and cleanliness of the facilities. Furthermore, patients were given a full and detailed explanation of the way to get any concerns or complaints addressed.

The Patient's Charter and, more latterly, the NHS Plan [2] have further empowered patients within the national health system. This change within health has mirrored that which has occurred generally within society over the same period.

A culture of blame and litigation

There has been a sea change in society's attitude to individual responsibility over the past 50 years. From the stoicism arising from poverty and war, education and wealth has developed a culture in which accountability and compensation predominate. The enormous control which technology has now given the modern world over the environment in which we live, has created this culture. Without control, there is always an element of chance. Modern society is no longer comfortable with the concept that life is subject to risk, chance and luck.

Every company or organisation now has a customer complaints department and insurance companies are everywhere. Society encourages individuals to insure themselves against every potentiality and to seek recompense for every adverse event, whoever is at fault. This culture of accountability and compensation, added to an increased awareness, education and belief in modern medicine, has an enormous impact on the health services. Patients with the ability to recognise a quality service are now fully empowered to extend this recognition further and to demand quality on their own terms.

Redefining quality

Historically, quality patient care has been defined by those responsible for delivering it. As experts in their field, it was assumed that health professionals both understood, and aspired to, the provision of quality patient care. Of course they did, and still do. But so many things have now changed, both professionally and socially, that patients are no longer content with the definitions of quality that the professionals provide.

Health professionals would generally define quality care in terms of timely and thorough investigation, accurate diagnosis and appropriate treatment and follow-up. Patients, on the other hand, are more likely to concentrate on the more transparent issues of communication and choice. An increasingly powerful public is now demanding that health services accept and include these new definitions of quality care within the service that they provide.

The NHS modernisation programme does just this. By voting in a government that has been willing to act on the public's behalf, patients now have a National Health Service with a statutory duty to provide and demonstrate quality in care. If the government is unable to deliver the kind of health service that the country wants, the public will respond in the ballot box.

References

1   The Patient's Charter for England. Available at www.doh.gov.uk/pcharter.
2   The NHS Plan. A plan for investment. A plan for reform. Secretary of State for Health. HMSO, London, July 2000. Available at www.doh.gov.uk/nhsplan.

Further reading

- Your Guide to the NHS. www.nhs.uk/nhsguide.
- O'Neill O. A Question of Trust. BBC Reith Lectures 2002. www.bbc.co.uk/radio4.
- NHS Executive. Patient and public involvement in the new NHS. Department of Health, Leeds, 1999.
- Ham C, Alberti KGMM. The medical profession, the public, and the government. *BMJ* 2002; 324: 838-842.

Chapter 5

Quality and efficiency in health

Here is Pooh Bear, coming downstairs now, bump, bump, on the back of his head, behind Christopher Robin. It is, as far as he knows, the only way of coming downstairs, but sometimes he feels that there is really another way, if only he could stop bumping for a moment and think of it.
AA Milne

The shock waves that followed the announcement of the new quality agenda have resonated within the health service ever since. This has been in spite of many calls for change from within the service itself.

Many health professionals feel that this newest round of modernisation amounts simply to the latest set of hoops through which the NHS is required to jump. The jumping will continue for the duration that the hoops remain fashionable, or until the next big idea arrives on the scene. A further complaint has been that the health service is, once more, being pushed to fit into the rigid standards and processes of industry; processes which are simply not appropriate for such a complex area as health. And underlying all of this is a sense of bewilderment at the extent and the nature of the change now being demanded.

There is no doubt that dramatic upheaval is now upon us and that the road ahead is uncertain. The NHS has been through previous failed change processes in an attempt to increase the efficiency of healthcare provision and there is entrenched scepticism regarding further reorganisational efforts. These arguments against modernisation contain elements of both an apprehension of further disruption and an unwillingness to change. Those arguing that the NHS cannot be compared with other organisations might examine their own response to similar quality initiatives that have occurred in other public services. The police, education system and government themselves are increasingly brought to public account.

In order to gain a more sensible perspective on the current process of health modernisation, it is useful to consider the development of all quality initiatives. The tremendous social change that has occurred over the past 50 years has already been discussed. Its influence on both private and public business has been both profound and necessary.

Competition: quality and efficiency

Industry has always had to compete in a market environment and competition has always been based both on low cost and high quality. When faced with the international trading stage, major companies and international governments have had to work increasingly hard in order to compete successfully.

The quality initiatives now common to commercial industry originate from the industrial recovery following the Second World War. It was the Japanese who led the way on quality and efficiency in business. Faced with the enormity of regenerating their infrastructure and economy from the ravages of the war, they utilised United States (US) management experts and academics to begin to compete with the world dominant US corporations. Japanese industries then survived the spiralling wage costs and inflationary pressures of the 1970s oil crises better than those around them. This competitive edge established Japan as world leaders in quality management.

Risk management

From the 1970s onwards, both private and public organisations began to experience the impact of further social change. Aggressive trade unionism, increased litigation, equal opportunities and the radical effect of information technology meant that organisations were suddenly more exposed to legal, financial and political risk. Organisations therefore had to assess the cost and impact of any running errors that were made. Poor service reputation, wastage and inadequate productivity could all have a significant deleterious effect on business. The concept of risk management was born.

For industries on the sharp end of the competitive market, risk management was taken on board rapidly. Within non-complex industry the processes involved were fairly simple. But, even extremely complex industries such as the airlines introduced robust structures to protect them against potential phenomenal risk. For industries handling paying customers, risk management became a competitive necessity.

Public services also experienced increasing pressure to control labour costs and improve efficiency. But the pressure for change did not come simply from the public using the services provided. The public has never had direct power to remove its custom from public services, despite funding them through tax. The pressures for change within the public sector are more complex. They relate to public and media pressure as well as government policy and national and international market forces.

So what has happened in health? The 1983 Griffiths Report announced that the consensus management approach of the 1970s had not worked for the NHS. A new breed of manager or leader was needed to enable strong decision-making and to facilitate local change. NHS administration thus moved from a history of 'bureau-professionalism' to a new managerialism [1].

1989 NHS reforms

The origins of the 1989 NHS reforms lie in a political crisis of confidence in the late 1980s. The pressures on the then Conservative government were intense. The Confederation of British Industry pressured to keep labour costs down and to free up the economic market place. The public demanded a reduction in general taxation and improved choice in healthcare. Increasing numbers of high profile media cases continuously highlighted inadequate access to care caused by long-standing NHS inefficiencies. And at the same time there were enormous, and increasing, cost pressures from a rapidly ageing population and the inflationary costs of technological developments in healthcare. The escalating crisis forced a public promise by the Prime Minister, Margaret Thatcher, on the BBC's Panorama programme. She announced an intention to undertake and publish a fundamental review of the financing of the NHS.

But, it can be argued, the eventual outcome of Conservative plans for NHS reform altered neither the speed nor direction of the ship, but instead re-organised the fore and aft deckchairs to give a good view of the impending iceberg. Margaret Thatcher's government did not have the political heart to go back to square one and ask the radical political question: does the country still believe in an NHS that is comprehensive, free to all, and funded from general taxation?

The 1989 reforms, therefore, amounted simply to a review of the internal structure of the NHS. They devised the purchaser-provider split and introduced the political ideologies of promoting a market economy and internal competition into the NHS for the first time. It was intended that an internal market would drive out inefficiencies, improve choice and drive up quality.

The internal market

But the theory and practice of the internal market remained disconnected in all but a few peripheral areas. Fund-holding practices were able to force through a few service improvements in areas where it had been difficult to improve quality in the past. Hospitals began to compete but inevitably with some winners and some losers as a result. In this environment, integrated service planning became a strategic nightmare and patient choice was virtual, rather than a reality for most.

Placing the patient at the centre of the market might have been good in theory, but did not work in practice for two main reasons. First, the patient did not have the money to buy what they wanted since the money lay with the purchasing authorities. Second, despite increased education and information, the patient has never had full detailed professional knowledge of the types of service they might want or need. This knowledge lay with the health professional.

The third way

As a result of escalating dissatisfaction with healthcare, in 1997 the new Labour Government ended the internal market and replaced it with a 'third way' of collaborative market management. A firm intention to re-create an NHS that the public was by now demanding was backed by the announcement of real increases in funding.

This most recent modernisation programme aims at establishing strong, centrally led standards for services that inform and direct the local organisations which plan and modernise services. Formal measurement, monitoring and validation of standards are underwritten by a new statutory duty for quality in care. Continuous quality improvement has been placed squarely at the heart of the new NHS. And clinical governance is the mechanism through which modernisation will occur.

Clinical governance - a mechanism for change

But is clinical governance really any different from other quality initiatives? Table 1, adapted from Taylor [2], details just some of the many approaches which have been introduced over the last decade or more. There are some suggestions that clinical governance may be a new ball game altogether. Most notable, is the legal duty of quality of care that has been placed upon the NHS. Prior to the implementation of clinical governance, there was only one legal bottom line for a chief executive: to stay in budget. This has now been matched by a similar duty of quality of care: the new 'second bottom line'.

Furthermore, past quality initiatives have tended to be championed by one set of protagonists in the NHS, rather than by the service as a whole. When medical audit was introduced, it was the province of the doctors; quality assurance schemes tended to be promoted mainly by nurse managers and risk management schemes were predominantly financially driven. Thus, the centre ground for quality initiatives in the NHS over the last ten years has been more of a battleground, competed for by various professional factions. Clinical governance, with its concentration on multi-professional teamworking and evenly spread responsibility, has a chance of bringing some peace to this shared ground.

Clinical governance brings the opportunity for health professionals and managers to work towards a joint goal and on common ground with patients at the centre. The new quality initiative has arisen from service failure and what some see as a near fatal wounding in the relationship between the NHS and the patient. Rebuilding this relationship is of fundamental importance to health professionals and managers alike. If this can be done through improving the quality of care for patients, professionals and managers can work within one value that they truly share. An effective relationship between clinicians, managers and patients has to be developed if successful and worthwhile clinical governance is to have a chance of flourishing.

Moving forward

Thus, clinical governance has arisen from half a century of social, economic and healthcare change. And it has been presented to those within the NHS for a reason. The patients, whom we serve, have requested their place back on centre stage. Clinical governance is not a stick by which the health service is to be beaten, but a protective process which will benefit patients and health professionals alike.

There is little doubt that an organisation as unwieldy as the NHS is going to take a good deal of time to implement such quality change. But, Labour's modernisation programme has presented an opportunity for the health service to start re-meeting the demands of the public it serves. Furthermore, the NHS is being asked to strive for a principle in which it believes - quality in patient care. The question now is, how to do it?

Table 1. Quality initiatives in the NHS. *(Adapted and reproduced with the kind permission of the BMJ Publishing Group. Taylor D. Quality and professionalism in healthcare: a review of current initiatives in the NHS. BMJ 1996; 312: 626-9).*

Initiative / technique	Description
Accreditation systems	Techniques for assessing institutional fitness to practise.
Anticipated recovery pathways	Multi-disciplinary methods for planning and monitoring treatments.
Audit	Process for the systematic, cyclical review of the objectives and standards of practice.
Benchmarking/benchmarking clubs	Set of techniques for comparing processes between competitor organisations.
Business process re-engineering	Radical review of organisational activities, implemented using the methods of total quality management (TQM, see below).
BS 5750/ISO 9000	A form of accreditation based on review of documentation of standard operating processes.
Clinical audit	Multi-disciplinary, professionally led systematic review of patient care.
Clinical care pathways	An explicit guideline that identifies the ideal 'journey' for a patient (usually with a common problem) across care sectors and professional boundaries.
Clinical governance	A system of steps and procedures adopted by the NHS to ensure that patients receive the highest possible quality of care.
Cochrane Centre	Part of the NHS research and development programme; it organises systematic reviews of randomised controlled trials and other evidence of the effectiveness of clinical care.
Communications programmes	Good communications between providers of services and all their internal (same organisation) and external customers.
Complaints systems	The facilitation and analysis of customer complaints.
Consumer surveys	Large numbers of surveys and monitoring exercises, of varying quality, have been conducted by NHS agencies since 1990.
Disease management	Term commonly applied to healthcare quality management initiatives funded or run by the pharmaceutical industry. Also linked to the US term 'managed care'.
Effective Health Care Bulletins	Summary bulletins produced as a part of the research and development programme's push towards evidence-based care.
Evidence-based care	The promotion of clinical care practices based on good research evidence.
External probity and VFM (value for money) audit	Includes NHS studies such as those commissioned by the Audit Commission. External audits may have either or both policing and developmental functions.

Table 1. Quality initiatives in the NHS. *contd:-*

Initiative / technique	Description
Health Quality Survey	A form of accreditation and linked developmental support run by the King's Fund and allied organisations (previously known as King's Fund Organisational Audit).
Inspectorates	Public service health and welfare inspectorates including the Commission for Health Improvement and the Audit Commission.
Medical/uni-professional audit	Clinical audit that is undertaken within a single professional discipline.
Modernisation	The term used within the Labour Government's NHS Plan to represent a radical approach to re-engineering health services.
National Service Frameworks	Published national standards for NHS service delivery in key priority areas eg. diabetes, older people.
National Institute for Clinical Excellence	A special Health Authority set up in 1999 to provide patients, health professionals and the public with authoritative, robust and reliable guidance on current best clinical practice.
Patient's Charter	A set of monitored patient rights and standards first established in 1992 as part of the Conservative government's Citizen's Charter initiative.
Patient focus	An approach originally developed by US management consultants, designed to ensure that patients' 'journeys' through care processes are timely and convenient.
Performance indicators and targets	As contained, for example, in the Health of the Nation programme.
Protocols/guidelines	Sets of treatment options and agreed decision making criteria, which may serve as a basis for systematic evaluation of clinical and allied care standards.
Quality of life measurement	There are now over 400 English language instruments available for assessing quality of life, either in relation to specific conditions or overall wellbeing.
Quality management assessment systems	A form of organisational audit. Examples include the Malcolm Baldrige award in the US and the European Quality Award.
Risk management	An approach to quality improvement based on techniques designed to minimise the risk of unwanted events for which the organisation might be liable or otherwise incur costs.
Total quality management	TQM techniques seek to enhance organisational sensitivity to customer requirements and optimally involve everyone in an organisation in meeting them.

References

1   Clarke J, Newman J. *The Managerial State: power, politics and ideology in the remaking of social welfare*. Sage, London, 1997.

2   Taylor D. Quality and professionalism in healthcare: a review of current initiatives in the NHS. *BMJ* 1996; 312: 626-9.

Further reading

•   Secretary of State for Health. A First Class Service. Department of Health, London, 1998.

•   Scally G, Donaldson LJ. Clinical governance and the drive for quality improvement in the new NHS in England. *BMJ* 1998; 317: 61-65.

•   A commitment to quality, a quest for excellence. Department of Health, London, 2001.

•   The A-Z of quality. NHS Management Executive, Leeds, 1993.

•   Berwick DM. Continuous improvement as an ideal in healthcare. *N Engl J Med* 1989; 320: 53-56.

PART II

Defining clinical governance

The launch of clinical governance presented us all with the chance to demonstrate that our fingers were on the political pulse. Here was a name that could be dropped with effect but, rather like the latest schoolyard slang, with the slight concern that it might be embarrassing to have to explain exactly what it meant! The chapters in Part II try to clarify what is meant by clinical governance and set out who has what role in delivering this agenda.

Chapter 6

Introducing clinical governance

"When I use a word", Humpty Dumpty said, in rather a scornful tone, "it means just what I choose it to mean - neither more nor less."
"The question is", said Alice, "whether you can make words mean so many different things."
Lewis Carroll

Having swept to power in May 1997, the newly elected Labour Government quickly published its vision of a new health service with quality of care for patients at its heart. *The New NHS - Modern and Dependable* heralded an end to the internal market and the pretence of financial competition that had been a feature of health policy under 20 years of conservative government. Tony Blair promised a new age [1].

> "Creating the NHS was the greatest act of modernisation ever achieved by a Labour Government. It banished the fear of becoming ill that had for years blighted the lives of millions of people. But I know that one of the main reasons people elected a new Government on May 1st was their concern that the NHS was failing them and their families. In my contract with the people of Britain I promised that we would rebuild the NHS."

Clinical governance - a new concept or just repackaging?

The term 'clinical governance' was first introduced in *The New NHS - Modern and Dependable*. It was introduced as:

"A new initiative .... to assure and improve clinical standards at local level throughout the NHS. This includes action to ensure that risks are avoided, adverse events are rapidly detected, openly investigated and lessons learned, good practice is rapidly disseminated and systems are in place to ensure continuous improvements in clinical care."

The term governance itself was not new. In the early 1990s, after the publication of the Cadbury Report [2], the business world was being driven to improve its corporate governance. The public sector, including the NHS, was following suit. The aim was to create a system in which an organisation could be directed and controlled to achieve its objectives and meet the necessary standards of accountability, probity and openness. This specified the need for accountability to be held at a senior management level. The introduction of clinical governance in the NHS in 1997 was therefore only a natural extension of this earlier work to ensure better control over the core business of the NHS - that of caring for patients. The cloak of governance has spread even further now to embrace both research governance and information governance. All of these concepts share the common theme of creating better systems to ensure objectives are achieved more consistently and with better overall quality.

Virtual reality

Following the debut of clinical governance in 1997, under the personal leadership of the government's newly appointed Chief Medical Officer - Liam Donaldson, flesh was put on the bones of the concept. Within the year, the document *A First Class Service: Quality in the new NHS* was published and famously defined clinical governance as:

"A framework through which NHS organisations are accountable for continuously improving the quality of their services and safeguarding high standards of care by creating an environment in which excellence in clinical care will flourish."

Working within the clinical governance framework was now a formal and explicit statutory duty for every part of the health service. For the very first time, chief executives within the NHS would be legally accountable for their organisation complying with this responsibility.

But it was still a concept that the NHS had to transform into a reality.

Putting theory into practice

Since the publication of *A First Class Service: Quality in the new NHS* there have been considerable efforts made at the clinical coalface to put theory into practice. Many within the NHS have struggled to understand this new concept. Not surprisingly an industry of articles, books (like this one!) and management consultancy has sprung up to guide the bemused clinician through the quality maze.

The problems of understanding lay not so much in what was presented, but to a greater extent in what had not been said. The introduction of an explicit patient-centred quality initiative into the health service was generally welcomed. No-one could argue with the intent. But how was it to be done and what did it actually mean in practice? To what extent is clinical governance merely a repackaging of the existing ways that clinicians assure the quality of what they do, for example through clinical audit and guideline development? These questions still remain, in some clinicians' eyes, unanswered.

Since 1997, an enormous amount of effort has been put into making clinical governance as a concept, both understandable and user friendly. A number of Commission for Health Improvement (CHI) published reports on NHS Trusts have noted the successful implementation and ownership of clinical governance at a corporate strategic board level. But what about lower down the organisational hierarchy? To what extent has clinical governance properly diffused down to clinicians at the grassroots in terms of better ways of working? Managers, doctors and senior nurses now have a greater familiarity with the phraseology of clinical governance [3] but practical demonstrations of implementation at the patient interface remain patchy rather than truly widespread. CHI has recognised this fact in its scoring systems used when reviewing NHS organisations (see page 45).

Definitions

In an attempt to simplify the concept for those trying to get to grips with it themselves (or indeed teaching others), we have gathered a few of the more user-friendly definitions of the clinical governance process:

Definitions of clinical governance

◆ A framework for the improvement of patient care through commitments to high standards, reflective practice, risk management and personal and team development [4].

◆ A clear framework for the achievement of quality improvement [5].

◆ Corporate accountability for clinical performance [6].

◆ The means by which organisations ensure the provision of quality clinical care by making individuals accountable for setting, maintaining and monitoring performance standards [7].

◆ The expectations and responsibilities on individuals and organisations to put in place systems which ensure the delivery of high quality healthcare [8].

We wonder if the search for the holy grail definition is really that important. Most writers on the subject acknowledge that the core of clinical governance seems to be centred on an individual's attitudes to personal and corporate accountability, patient care and professional responsibilities. The specific management skills and techniques that are needed in order to make individual aspects of clinical governance work are of secondary importance.

References

1   The New NHS, Modern, Dependable. Secretary of State for Health. The Stationery Office, London, December 1997.

2   Report of the Committee on The Financial Aspects of Corporate Governance. 1 December 1992. Gee and Co. Ltd.
    Available at www.ecgi.org/codes/country_documents/uk/cadbury.pdf.

3   Firth-Cozens J. Clinical governance development needs in health service staff. *Clinical Performance & Quality Health Care* 1999; 7(4):155-60.

4   Clinical governance: practical advice for primary care in England and Wales. RCGP, January 1999.

5   Clinical governance in the New NHS. British Association of Medical Managers, 1998.

6   Unattributed.

7   Clinical governance in North Thames: a draft paper for discussion and consultation. Department of Public Health and Strategy, NHSE North Thames Regional Office. 1998.

8   Dunning M, Ayres P. What is clinical governance? A workable definition. *Healthcare Quality* 1998; 4(3):16-18.

Further reading

• Scally G, Donaldson LJ. Clinical governance and the drive for quality improvement in the new NHS in England. *BMJ* 1998; 317: 61-65.

• Clinical governance: Quality in the new NHS. NHS Executive, London, 1999. (HSC 1999/065).

• Your own Trust's last CHI report. www.chi.nhs.uk/eng/organisations/index.shtml.

• Governance in the NHS. NHS Executive, London, 1999. (HSC 1999/123).

Chapter 7

Clinical governance in the workplace

Beauty is altogether in the eye of the beholder.
Margaret Wolfe Hungerford

Whose measure of quality?

Before we can tackle the nitty-gritty of any quality assurance process like clinical governance we have to know what we mean by 'quality'. As we discussed in Chapter 5 this is the basis of any industry - to do the job properly and to the highest standard.

Quality in the NHS

The oft quoted definition of quality in the NHS [1] is doing the:
◆ right thing in the
◆ right way at the
◆ right time and for the
◆ right patient

Clinical governance describes the systems that we must put in place to help us achieve this.

Getting the quality balance right

For the manufacturing industry, creating quality standards is relatively straightforward. Widget production has some straightforward (and measurable) outcomes. But within any service industry (eg. healthcare, education, social services), of course, there is a catch. Each person passing through the process is individual and often unpredictable. As well as this, the needs of individuals are frequently complex. Therefore, the patient or client often has to access services across many different providers on a multitude of levels, any of which may not live up to their expectations of quality.

In the NHS, definitions of quality have tended to be driven by those commissioning and providing care, that is, managers and clinicians. In other sectors, where the customer is the payer, quality is often concerned more with the way in which services are provided. Good communication and customer comfort are typically deemed to be of great importance. Somehow a balance needs to be struck in healthcare between the different agendas of the provider and the consumer. The clinical governance standpoint is that these two perspectives are both valid and significant.

The ten commandments of clinical governance

With a broad definition of quality understood as the basis for good clinical care, what are the components that we need to have in place in our hospitals, departments and professional lives to ensure safe, effective and up-to-date care? Terms such as strategic direction, ownership and learning effectiveness make little constructive sense to professionals not brought up to be comfortable with a mindset of management processes and jargon. Far more effective is to think of the components of clinical governance in terms of current systems that we have already in place to some degree or other.

The ten commandments or components of clinical governance were described originally in *A First Class Service: Quality in the NHS* [2] (see facing page).

Failing current systems

So perhaps we should now feel reassured that most of this activity is already being undertaken to some extent or another. Many of the

The ten commandments of clinical governance

A quality organisation will ensure that:

◆ quality improvement processes (eg. clinical audit) are in place and integrated with the quality programme for the organisation as a whole.

◆ leadership skills are developed at clinical team level.

◆ evidence-based practice is in day-to-day use with the infrastructure to support it.

◆ good practice, ideas and innovations (which have been evaluated) are systematically disseminated within and outside the organisation.

◆ clinical risk reduction programmes of a high standard are in place.

◆ adverse events are detected, and openly investigated; and the lessons learned promptly applied.

◆ lessons for clinical practice are systematically learned from complaints made by patients.

◆ problems of poor clinical performance are recognised at an early stage and dealt with to prevent harm to patients.

◆ all professional development programmes reflect the principles of clinical governance.

◆ the quality of data collected to monitor clinical care is itself of a high standard.

structures and systems required are already in place. Each NHS Trust already has departments managing audit, risk, clinical incidents, complaints and data collection. Every Trust will also have professional development programmes in place along with staff disciplinary procedures.

However, the whole seems to add up to less than the sum of its parts! Why, despite all of these systems already in place, do we still have unacceptable variations in clinical care and a public with decreasing confidence in the way we assure quality of care?

What doesn't help is the lack of co-ordinated working within organisations. Examples of good practice may abound but, because they tend not to be shared and disseminated, their value is automatically limited.

Causes of variations in clinical care

◆ Departments and individuals working in isolation.
◆ Rigid professional boundaries and territorialism.
◆ Lack of agreed protocols of care/care pathways across departments and organisations.
◆ Inadequate time and practical support to help clinical teams reflect on and change their practice.

The need to communicate

Consider the issue of clinical risk management. How effective are the links between risk managers, the clinical audit department and the consultant body in the average NHS Trust? The chances are that the hospital clinical audit programme is driven by clinicians' own interests and not necessarily by what the hospital corporately sees as its main clinical risk areas. Clinical governance emphasises the need for the left and right hand to know what each is doing and ultimately influence each other positively. Simple and effective communication therefore is critical.

However, improving communication about quality issues within the NHS is not sufficient; there is seen to be a need to engage with the public at large to a far greater degree than has been the practice to date. One of the reasons why a firm political grip has been taken on driving clinical governance in the NHS, has been because of the perceived loss of public confidence in the service. The use of NHS league tables and 'starring' of NHS Trusts are examples of government attempts at demonstrating any improvement in NHS performance and reductions in the variations in quality of care.

The success of clinical governance therefore will likely be measured in political terms by the strength of public confidence in the NHS. Communicating with the public on what we do and how we perform is now an essential feature of the work of healthcare organisations. At its worst this might be regarded as a political gimmick, open to cynical manipulation for political gain. However, there is the counter argument that openness and public involvement in the systems we have in place in our hospitals and surgeries, is beneficial to us all.

References

1   Clinical Effectiveness Steering Group Report. Royal College of Nursing. London. RCN 1996a.

2   A First Class Service. Quality in the new NHS. Secretary of State for Health. Department of Health, London, 1998.

Further reading

•   Halligan A, Donaldson L. Implementing clinical governance: turning vision into reality. *BMJ* 2001; 322: 1413-1417.

Chapter 8

Whose responsibility is clinical governance?

The buck stops here. **Harry S Truman**
The buck stops with the guy who signs the cheques. **Rupert Murdoch**

Everyone's business

Where does responsibility for clinical governance lie in the NHS? The oft-quoted aphorism that "clinical governance is everyone's business" is a truism but different aspects of clinical governance work can be seen at all levels within an organisation. In this chapter we look at the different roles from Trust Board level to the clinical team and finally the individual clinician.

The Trust Board

The second bottom line

For many years all a hospital chief executive had to worry about was balancing the books and solving the perennial hospital car parking problem. As an accountable officer the chief executive was responsible before Parliament for the 'stewardship of resources' within the Trust.

But clinical governance changed all this. As well as a statutory duty for financial stewardship, the chief executive and the Board now has a statutory duty in relation to quality. In other words the chief executive must put and keep in place arrangements for monitoring and improving the quality of the healthcare that is provided by the Trust - the so-called 'second bottom line'.

Power to ensure this duty of care of course, relies heavily on having the right processes in place to enable good clinical governance to happen.

Because measuring valid outcomes of patient care is still an elusive goal in the NHS, except perhaps when there has been an obvious serious lapse of care, the focus and responsibility for the Trust Board is to demonstrate it has the right processes and systems in place.

Establishing Trust systems for clinical governance

Trusts are required to have in place solid processes for successful clinical governance. The Trust should be able to demonstrate:

- clear lines of responsibility and accountability through having:
  - ➤ *a designated board-level senior clinician responsible for clinical governance, usually the Medical Director.*
  - ➤ *a clinical governance sub-committee chaired by a Board non-executive reporting to the Board on a monthly basis.*
  - ➤ *a clinical governance development programme and annual public report on progress on what the Trust is doing to assure quality.*
- participation in a CHI review every four years, implementing the recommendations and action points raised in the review.
- implementation of National Institute for Clinical Excellence (NICE) guidelines.
- collection (and submission centrally) of data to monitor and review clinical performance.

Trust star ratings

NHS organisations are to be 'star-rated' in the near future independently of government. The Commission for Health Improvement (CHI) is to merge with part of the Audit Commission (and the National

Care Standards Commission) to create the new Commission for Healthcare Audit & Inspection (CHAI) to take on this assessment role. They will use a 'balanced scorecard' approach. This approach attempts to develop an overall star rating for each Trust based on a broad range of indicators. Some of these indicators are given stronger weighting than others eg. access to services.

Trusts with top scores of three stars will be granted 'earned autonomy' eg. less in-depth performance management by the new Strategic Health Authorities. They will also be eligible to apply for foundation hospital status with even greater freedoms proposed.

Measuring Trust clinical performance

Despite the problems of using indicators to measure accurately how a Trust performs, it is still a reality. The indicators that are used in star rating Trusts are assessed across six areas known as the NHS performance assessment framework.

The national performance assessment framework focuses on six areas (see facing page), selected to capture "what really counts for patients and for staff". The success of the new NHS is to be judged in-part on whether it makes improvements across all aspects of this framework[1].

Within the framework there are a number of specific clinical outcome indicators used to make local and national comparisons between similar Trusts [2]. These contribute to the overall star rating of Trusts (see page 44).

CHI reviews

CHI (and CHAI later) aim to review all NHS organisations, by looking at their clinical governance systems and overall quality of care, every few years. Readers who have been involved in their own Trust's CHI review, will know how detailed and demanding the process can be for all concerned. Following the review, an action plan to address significant weaknesses is developed by the Trust and agreed with CHI and the relevant Strategic Health Authority.

Six dimensions of the NHS performance assessment framework

◆ **Health improvement** (i.e. reflecting the overall aim of improving the general health of the population, influenced by many factors reaching well beyond the NHS).
  ➢ *For example, changes in rates of premature death, reflecting social and economic factors as well as healthcare.*

◆ **Fair access** (i.e. recognising that the NHS must offer fair access to health services in relation to people's needs, irrespective of geography, class, ethnicity, age or sex).
  ➢ *For example, ensuring that black and minority ethnic groups are not disadvantaged in terms of access to services.*

◆ **Effective delivery of appropriate healthcare** (i.e. recognising that care must be effective, appropriate, timely and complies with agreed standards).
  ➢ *For example, increasing provision of treatments proven to bring benefit such as hip replacements, provision of rehabilitation at the point when it can offer most benefit, sustained delivery of health and social care to those with long-term needs, and reducing inappropriate treatments.*

◆ **Efficiency** (i.e. the way in which the NHS uses its resources to achieve value for money).
  ➢ *For example, length of hospital stay; day surgery rates; unit costs; labour productivity; management overheads; capital productivity.*

◆ **Patient and carer experience** (i.e. measuring the way in which patients and carers view the quality of the treatment and care that they receive, ensuring the NHS is sensitive to individual needs).
  ➢ *For example, percentage of those on the waiting list waiting 12 months or more, delayed discharge from hospital for those aged 75 or over.*

◆ **Health outcomes of NHS care** (i.e. assessing the direct contribution of NHS care to improvements in overall health, completing the circle back to the overarching goal of improved health).
  ➢ *For example, trends in infectious diseases for which immunisation programmes are available.*

Clinical outcome indicators for Trust comparisons

♦ Deaths within 30 days of surgery (elective admissions).
♦ Deaths within 30 days of a heart bypass operation.
♦ Deaths within 30 days of admission with a hip fracture.
♦ Deaths within 30 days of admission with a stroke.
♦ Emergency readmission to hospital within 28 days of discharge.
♦ Emergency readmission to hospital within 28 days of discharge following treatment for a fractured hip.
♦ Emergency readmission to hospital within 28 days of discharge following treatment for a stroke.
♦ Discharge to usual place of residence within 56 days of emergency admission from there, with a stroke.
♦ Discharge to usual place of residence within 28 days of emergency admission from there, with a hip fracture.

We do not intend in this book to go into the detail of how a CHI review is conducted. It is useful, however, to note that CHI looks at seven key component areas during their review process.

CHI review areas

♦ Patient and public involvement.
♦ Clinical audit.
♦ Risk management.
♦ Clinical effectiveness programmes.
♦ Staffing and staff management.
♦ Education, training and continuing personal and professional development.
♦ Use of information to support clinical governance and healthcare delivery.

By looking at these areas they are also assessing two key aspects: the patient experience and the Trust's strategic capacity for developing and implementing clinical governance.

On the basis of the evidence collected, CHI assesses each of the seven components of clinical governance above against a four-point scale.

> ### CHI's scale for assessing each component of clinical governance
>
> ◆ **I** = little or no progress at strategic and planning level, or at operational level.
> ◆ **IIa** = worthwhile progress and development at strategic and planning levels but not at operational level or,
> **IIb** = worthwhile progress and development at operational level but not at strategic and planning levels or,
> **IIc** = worthwhile progress and development at strategic and planning levels and at operational level but not across the whole organisation.
> ◆ **III** = good strategic grasp and substantial implementation. Alignment across the strategic and planning levels, and the operational level of the Trust.
> ◆ **IV** = excellence - co-ordinated activity and development across the organisation and with partner organisations in the local health economy that is demonstrably leading to improvement. Clarity about the next stage of clinical governance

These scores are used during the star ratings assessment for the Trust. In this way a Trust doing very well on the performance indicators can still fall foul of a top three star rating through poor CHI review scores.

The change of organisational title from the Commission for Health Improvement to the Commission for Healthcare Audit & Inspection is for some a subtle but nonetheless radical change in their role in assuring the quality of care in the NHS.

Working together

As well as the Trust's responsibilities internally to promote better standards of care, it also has a duty to work in partnership with other NHS organisations. Working closely with Primary Care Trusts in developing their Local Delivery Plans (LDPs) is part of this.

The days of an NHS Trust acting in splendid isolation without regard for other NHS partners are over. As well as information on progress against service agreements, NHS Trusts are now required to make available their annual operating plans and regular reports on progress against them to their local Primary Care Trusts. Important investment decisions, for example, in new high tech equipment, or in a new consultant post, will need to be consistent with the local LDPs.

The clinical team

Linking clinicians into systems

Having looked at the Trust's organisational role and responsibility in clinical governance, it would be normal now to consider the role and responsibility of the individual clinician. We believe, however, the clinical team/unit or department is also an important structure in delivering effective clinical governance.

The department acts as the link between the internal processes set up by the Trust and the professional responsibilities of the practising clinician. It encourages a multi-disciplinary approach to the implementation of clinical governance and in most cases provides a more comfortable and practical environment for concerns to be raised and discussed. It has to be recognised that some readers may doubt that this is the case when they look at their own clinical team dynamics!

Valuing differences

The importance of multi-disciplinary working in clinical governance cannot be overstated. Other clinicians see the patient experience in different ways so that it is useful to recognise the differing range of skills that individual clinicians bring to the bedside. Communication skills are obviously vital but other multi-disciplinary skills include the ability to interpret information, to manage clinical uncertainty and to systematise care.

Professional attitudes also vary across disciplines. A medicalised view of the patient/liver/lung in the bed needs to be balanced with the more holistic approach to patient care that is favoured by nursing colleagues.

Team work

From a practical point of view, the clinical department usually offers a sensible organisational level for the arrangement of clinical governance meetings and discussions on risk management, critical incidents, case management, training and education, audit projects and the planning of appraisal systems.

Specific national targets such as two-week cancer waits can often be more easily tackled using departmental discussion and planning rather than by imposing a whole-Trust solution. A further example might be a department's strategy for trying to achieve Cancer Unit or Centre status; reaching such targets depends on a strong and consistent team effort.

All of this departmental activity on clinical governance requires one essential component - that of time. A well organised and motivated department can make a case for planned quality time within the working week with the support of unit managers.

The clinician

Clinical governance - an opportunity?

Finally we consider the role of the practising clinician. It would be easy and understandable for clinicians to reject the notion of clinical governance as an imposed and unnecessary management initiative. This would be an unfortunate and perhaps ill-considered response. We believe that clinical governance offers each healthcare professional an opportunity to improve morale and regain a measure of control over professional development and standards of care.

The national professional regulatory bodies have realised the sea change that is upon us and have re-emphasised the critical importance of setting and promoting standards. The onus now falls on clinicians to ensure they rise to these standards - by keeping competencies up-to-date and by maintaining individual professional registration.

The responsibilities of each healthcare professional in terms of clinical governance are implied, rather than listed as statutory duties as they have been for the Trust. We are each responsible for ensuring that quality is at the core of the service that we provide. Appraisal, professional development plans, revalidation and training needs assessment will become as familiar to doctors over the next decade as the use of computers in medicine has been over the last.

A reality check

When brought to a practical level this means understanding the nature of our jobs and doing them well. This makes sense and no-one would argue with the intent. However, reality within the NHS today is all too often a far cry from the simplicity of such a statement.

There are numerous examples of the disparity between what each of us knows to be good practice, and the reality of the normal working environment within a Trust. The box on the facing page highlights just a few of these.

None of this will be new to any moderately experienced health professional and many will wonder why more extreme examples have not been chosen. Everyday examples are valuable as an aid to pointing out that healthcare professionals work with a constant dilemma within the modern NHS, day-in and day-out. Does the patient before us in the outpatient department/on the ward/in casualty, get the time and attention

The poor quality realities of NHS practice

◆ The pretence that ward curtains are soundproof.
◆ Excessive waiting times throughout the service.
◆ Absence of staff to sit with patients given bad news.
◆ Time limitations on patient discussions with doctors.
◆ Last minute cancellations of surgical procedures.
◆ Reviewing patients in clinic without their medical notes.

that they require both physically and emotionally whilst others wait? Or do we attempt to provide all of the patients before us with a safe, yet basic service - a Rolls Royce or Ford NHS?

As individuals we have very little guidance on this and many varying opinions abound on each issue. For example, when we see patients in clinic without notes, we would all concede that this is a potentially dangerous practice and certainly does not constitute a quality service. But what options do we have? We can refuse to see any patient whose notes are not available on the basis of dangerous practice, we can see the patient without their notes ensuring that we have documented the absence of the notes, or we can rely on already busy clinic staff to search for the notes, recent investigation results or past clinic letters. Each of us will know people who tackle this situation in different ways. But which is the right way?

Until such a time that we are given clear guidance on the correct way to tackle this type of situation, each of us must make an informed choice of how we provide a quality service to our patients within the limits of our surroundings.

Personal responsibilities

There are certain things that we can do. As individuals we can accept responsibility for our contributions to team working and understand that we are individually responsible for ensuring that our part of any care is undertaken with the patient's well-being as paramount. We also have a responsibility to ensure we expand our understanding on issues such as patient consent, communication and documentation, as well as familiarising ourselves with relevant NICE guidance and published National Service Frameworks (NSFs).

Finally, we have a shared responsibility for team colleagues in supporting them should they be having problems professionally or personally. However, it is also clear that hiding our heads in the sand, when a colleague is known to be under-performing, is a serious breach of professional standards on our part. We return later in the book to consider this important issue in more detail under the topic of risk management.

References

1   8.5: The New NHS, Modern, Dependable. Secretary of State for Health. December 1997. The Stationery Office, London, 1997.
2   6.0: The New NHS, Modern, Dependable. Secretary of State for Health. December 1997. The Stationery Office, London, 1997.

Further reading

• NHS Performance Indicators: A Consultation. Principles of Developing and Using Performance Indicators (Annex 5). www.doh.gov.uk/piconsultation/principles.htm.
• Your own Trust's last CHI report. www.chi.nhs.uk/eng/organisations/index.shtml.
• CHI's guidelines for NHS organisations preparing for a review. www.chi.nhs.uk/eng/cgr/index.shtml.
• Emerging themes from 175 CHI reviews. www.chi.nhs.uk/eng/cgr/emerging_themes.pdf.

PART III

Practical considerations

Part III examines some of the basic materials which are essential requirements if clinical governance-driven change is to take place. Healthcare is awash with data, but there are significant dangers in collecting and using flawed or misinterpreted information. However, while data accumulates, time drifts away; there can be few individuals working within the NHS who do not feel pressure on their time. If quality improvement is to continue at an optimum pace, time is a resource that must be valued and used intelligently. Finally, the skills and techniques of project management are discussed. Without effective project management many well-intentioned efforts are likely to end in frustration and failure.

Chapter 9

Data quality & confidentiality

Where is the wisdom we have lost in knowledge?
Where is the knowledge we have lost in information?
T S Eliot

There was a time, no more than ten years ago, when arguments could be won and decisions made on the basis of professional opinion alone. That era has passed, and has been replaced by one within which information and data are seen as vital components which are essential to future planning. However, the Holy Grail of a truly evidence-based healthcare system has not yet been reached. The shortfall is down to the remaining gaps in medical knowledge and the poor quality of much of our data. Furthermore, data analysis and interpretation remains, all too often, critically flawed.

Information is powerful and when appropriately applied can be highly beneficial. But the power of poorly applied or misinterpreted data is also potentially dangerous. The introduction of league tables into the public services illustrates both the benefits and pitfalls of information use. In education for example, parents use league tables to identify schools with good examination records. However, there will always be some schools in relatively deprived areas; despite performing well for their students these schools may still find themselves well down the examination league table, and appear to be failing. It is therefore obvious that raw data need to be correctly analysed and interpreted in context if their beneficial effects are to be released.

The importance and power of information has not been lost on those who have been charged with developing NHS modernisation. A national

Information Strategy (Information for Health) was published in 1998 [1]. Its ambitious scope includes the development of a comprehensive NHS electronic network, the introduction of electronic patient records, the standardisation of information (such as the use of Read codes) and the development of the National Electronic Library for Health. Of particular interest is the plan to provide all healthcare professionals with online access to evidence and guidance, along with the necessary support to allow evaluation of their own service and professional development.

Evidently, effective service evaluation and professional assessment can only be locally performed with the use of accurate and recent data. But, the modern hunger for information can also make us short-sighted. On occasion, enormous effort is put into data collection whilst neglecting to ascertain whether or not the data collected will be capable of generating information that is going to be interpretable and useful.

Data collection

An illustration of the need for a questioning approach to data collection can be drawn from the cancer registration service which has been established in the UK for over 40 years. The network of Cancer Registries contains the most accurate and complete cancer statistics in the world. However, some may argue that the clinical benefits derived from this resource do not justify the major investment made. Others will point to the significant opportunities in cancer audit and epidemiological research provided by such rich data sources. It is therefore difficult to assess fully the cost-benefits of the cancer registry network from the differing perspectives of patient, clinician, researcher and health service planner.

Despite these concerns, there is no doubt that all clinical departments should be collecting data. However, the process must not be passive and unplanned. A data strategy is always needed, even if the strategy is relatively informal. Perhaps the crucial step in improving data management is to carry out a critical review of current data-collection activity and to prioritise these efforts. By assessing the information collected both by an individual department and by the wider organisation, the resources going into data collection will be highlighted. Manpower and information technology are most effectively targeted once the whole picture is clear.

Clinical input and control is essential to effective research and audit data. In contrast, much of the routine performance data that is collected should be independent of clinical input once the mechanism of collection has been devised and clerical staff have been trained. There will always be areas of overlap where some ongoing clinical input may be mutually beneficial. For example, clinical coding is demanded by the performance management agenda and, if accurately performed, may provide a valuable audit and research resource.

Practical suggestions

- Make sure you know the types of information which are currently being collected within your unit.
- Analyse the value of the information in a critical way - who is it for, what is the purpose of its collection? Only put your departmental and personal efforts into data collection which is truly valuable.
- Make sure that the detail of the information collected is appropriate - don't waste time collecting data that are either too basic or unnecessarily detailed.
- Plan how data are to be analysed and what questions the information will be expected to answer prior to any data collection.
- Make sure that the people collecting data are adequately trained for the task.
- If there is a need for quality control arrangements, make sure they are in place.

Data storage

The advent of the personal computer has transformed our ability to store and handle data. With the increase in machine specification, software developments and miniaturisation, our data handling capabilities will continue to advance. Many of the pioneers of clinical audit were IT enthusiasts and such skills are now widespread within medical practice. Indeed, the European Computer Driving Licence (ECDL) is now the NHS reference standard for IT competence and free IT training is offered in many centres. There is therefore no excuse for storing data in a way which does not allow easy input, access and analysis. Those working within the NHS without the requisite skills for data storage and handling should always seek assistance and advice.

Practical suggestions

- Consider carefully whether data should be collected in a stand-alone system or with links into your organisation's IT networks.
- Store data within one of the industry standard database or spreadsheet formats in order to allow ease of manipulation.
- Maintain back-up copies of data.
- Work out what output will be needed from the data storage and ensure that the data will be sufficiently detailed to meet that need.
- Consider carrying out a power calculation to check that you will have enough information to draw sensible conclusions.
- Do not collect lots of information 'just in case' - it is likely to result in much wasted time and to clutter up the storage system.
- Try to avoid descriptive information that may not be amenable to interpretation or analysis when reviewed at a later date.
- Ensure compliance with confidentiality legislation.

Data protection and confidentiality

The 1984 Data Protection Act [2] put issues of data confidentiality under statutory control. Its foundation has been built on by further Parliamentary legislation which was enacted in 1998 [3]. The specific problems raised by patient-identifiable information within the NHS were examined by the Caldicott Committee, which reported in 1997 [4]. Human rights legislation is also likely to have an impact in this area. Healthcare workers have therefore been provided with considerable help and guidance with regard to data issues. In the modern climate all NHS staff must be aware of the potential for legal redress for individuals who suffer as a result of a breach in confidentiality.

1998 Data Protection Act

Requires registration by 'data controllers' thereby creating a register which is available to public scrutiny. Furthermore it sets out the principles of data protection, which include the following.

◆ The requirement to process data fairly and only if necessary.

◆ The requirement for a subject's consent, which must be explicit in the case of sensitive personal information.

◆ To use data only for the purposes for which it was obtained.

◆ To only collect data which is relevant and not excessive.

◆ To maintain data in an accurate and up-to-date manner.

◆ Not keeping data longer than is necessary for the original need.

◆ Maintaining safeguards to protect data confidentiality.

Caldicott and its impact

The introduction of a legal framework for information control had only resulted in a somewhat haphazard approach to issues of confidentiality and security in the NHS; the law may have been there but custom and practice was often the stronger influence. This was recognised by the Caldicott Committee who designed a strategy to improve on the operational information standards of the NHS, governing patient identifiable information.

The Caldicott Principles

1. Justify the purpose for using confidential information.
2. Only use it when absolutely necessary.
3. Use the minimum that is required.
4. Access should be on a strict need-to-know basis.
5. Everyone must understand his or her responsibilities.
6. Understand and comply with the law.

The chosen solution of the Caldicott Committee hinges on the work of Caldicott Guardians who are now appointed within all NHS organisations as well as Local Authority Social Service Departments.

The duties of a Caldicott Guardian

◆ Establishing local protocols for patient information disclosure.

◆ Introducing and enforcing arrangements for information access on a need-to-know principle.

◆ Setting up audit processes to monitor information pathways and use.

◆ Improving staff training, database design and other aspects of information handling.

◆ Introducing the Caldicott principles into clinical information management.

A Guardian is normally a Trust Board member and a senior health professional; their link with clinical governance structures must be demonstrated. Caldicott Guardians have a duty to oversee a number of developments in the field of patient information processing.

Data analysis

It is no accident that the concept of clinical governance has emerged at a time when evidence-based medicine has cemented the idea that the practice of medicine is a truly scientific endeavour. In every field of its activity, clinical governance demands evidence. However, data alone only provides us with information - correctly analysed data are the basis of evidence.

At present the NHS often falls short of its aspiration to be an organisation which is fundamentally evidence-based. It is extraordinary that, in some spheres, change depends on sophisticated research methodology and statistical analysis while, elsewhere in healthcare, meaningless, unprocessed data are accepted without question.

Numerical data generally require some element of statistical analysis in order to gauge impact. Medical education together with research experience now provides a good grounding in statistical techniques for many clinicians. However, higher-level statistical expertise is in frustratingly short supply within the NHS. Despite this limitation, healthcare professionals should be prepared to question the validity of data that have not been sensibly analysed. To do so is not a sign of academic arrogance, but demonstrates an interest in improving standards in this important area.

Practical suggestions

● If you are not confident about statistical methodology - consider how to fill the gap in your knowledge.

● Find out what statistical support is available within the Trust and make use of it.

● Undertake a power calculation before starting extensive data collection - can your question be satisfactorily answered by the information that is going to be gathered?

● Decide what level of proof you will need in order to act on a result of a data analysis eg. 95% confidence levels are usual in research but an audit might use less stringent criteria.

● Plan statistical analysis at the outset when starting a new project.

References

1   Information For Health - 1. An Information Strategy for the modern NHS. NHS Information Authority. Available at www.nhsia.nhs.uk.

2   The guidelines: The Data Protection Act 1984: using the law to protect your information. 3rd series. Office of the Data Protection Registrar, 1994.

3   Data Protection Act 1998. HMSO, July 1998.
     Available at www.legislation.hmso.gov.uk/acts/acts1998/19980029.htm.

4   The Caldicott Committee: Report on the review of patient-identifiable information. Department of Health, London, December 1997.
     Available at www.doh.gov.uk/ipu/confiden/report/caldrep.pdf.

Further reading

•   Building the Information Core: Implementing the NHS Plan. NHS Executive, Leeds, 2001.

•   Gardner MJ, Altman DG, eds. *Statistics with confidence*. BMJ Books, London, 1989.

Chapter 10

Quality time

Sometimes I sits and thinks, and then again I just sits.
Punch

For many years the inability of the NHS to match the expectations of the public and politicians has been put down, first and foremost, to a lack of financial investment. However, the importance of finance as the main limitation on NHS performance is now being challenged by the restrictions that are being imposed by difficulties with recruitment. More person-hours are needed to fulfil service commitments and meet performance targets. It is against this background that all healthcare professionals are feeling the pressure of a lack of time. The technical difficulties of a job may be challenging but the volume of work is all too often overwhelming. If clinical governance fails to deliver a quantum jump in the quality of healthcare, a shortage of professional time is likely to be a critical factor.

Time is a resource and should be regarded as such. Thus, peoples' time should be used appropriately. If there is a shortage of doctors it would seem sensible to provide additional administrative support so that clinical sessions run efficiently. All too often long waits to access a service go hand-in-hand with patients failing to attend when their name finally comes to the top of the list. Our current systems are not efficient.

Against this backdrop, it is interesting to note the extent of professional time that is consumed by some of the major quality initiatives. Audit was introduced amidst huge expectations of its power to deliver change and quality improvement. Clinical time was set aside on an unprecedented scale and yet that huge use of a scarce resource has not been subject to the level of scrutiny that financial expenditure receives. Similarly, we are now in the era of the cancer multi-disciplinary team meeting. Such gatherings are unarguably desirable but the question remains unanswered as to whether the clinical time that they so hungrily consume could be better invested.

Saving time

Good time management skills are essential for hard-pressed clinicians and managers. The encouragement to "work smarter not harder" may feel irritating and worn out but, infuriatingly, the concept remains relevant to most of us. The following tips are typical of the advice offered by time management trainers.

Practical suggestions

● Keep a prioritised 'to do' list. Keeping this record of tasks in hand helps time allocation and increases the chances of the jobs being completed.

● Maintain control over an efficient diary system.

● A weeklong log of your activities will demonstrate whether your time is being used effectively.

● Avoid unproductive meetings.

● Refuse excessive workloads; learn to say no.

● Set uninterrupted time aside for important tasks and avoid spending much effort on trivial jobs.

● Once started on a task, get it finished before moving on.

● Delegate frequently and effectively. Ensure that the subordinate understands the task and has the authority, knowledge and ability to carry it out.

● Maintain a balance between work, family life and recreation. Demands on one's time will be ever-present so that the balance can only be struck by making conscious efforts.

Making time

It is important to realise that the philosophy of clinical governance requires that time is set aside in order to attend to quality issues. This principle is well illustrated by the introduction of scheduled time for audit, which became established in the NHS in the 1990s. We therefore have a responsibility both to make time for clinical governance activities and to make good use of such time.

Many NHS Trusts will have a programme of half-day sessions that are cleared of routine clinical activity to enable audit and other clinical governance work to take place. There are many examples of excellent practice where this time is used to great effect. Unfortunately, in other areas, dreary and unproductive meetings fill these sessions - with subsequent poor attendance. With some thought and planning, it should be possible to make this time both useful and enjoyable.

Practical suggestions

- Widen the scope of clinical audit meetings to cover all aspects of clinical governance - don't be restricted to audit simply because that's how the sessions have been labelled.
- Ensure that at least some sessions are multi-disciplinary in both input and content.
- Vary the content to maintain interest. Gather ideas for the meeting agenda from other departments.
- Avoid routine data review unless it is definitely educational and interesting.
- Carry out a brief evaluation at the end of each session - what went well, what could be improved?
- Consider rotating the meeting chairmanship.

Routine sessions are undoubtedly valuable but some tasks and issues warrant more concentrated time and effort. Planning time-out is necessary if progress is to be made on complex problems or projects. If there is good justification for the use of this time then it is appropriate to sacrifice some clinical activity in order to make progress. Clinical governance provides a clear indication that service delivery cannot carry on in the absence of efforts to maintain the highest standards for that clinical work.

A further way in which the individual clinician can take some control over the quantity versus quality equation is in the scheduling of clinical work. A good example of this is the way in which the length of time given for individual General Practice consultations has been increasing. This has allowed for more effective doctor/patient contact but has the potential for increased waiting times for patients who are making appointments. The problem of access will need to be addressed but this is to be preferred to maintaining a failing pattern of clinical practice. The NHS has been full of examples where high throughput has been achieved by sacrificing quality standards. It is now clear that this trade-off is being reined in; clinicians are realising that high productivity is not necessarily a defence if things are seen to be going wrong.

Clinical governance contracts?

It is clear that clinical governance consumes time, energy and financial resources. The individual has clear responsibilities within this new agenda but can only meet these with the support of their Trust or organisation. One possible approach to clarifying the roles of the two parties is to formalise the process to some extent. Educational contracts have been in use for some years and a similar arrangement could be used within the re-accreditation process to aid clinical governance delivery. Indeed this was an explicit aspect of the proposed controversial new NHS consultant contract. All consultants were to have around three sessions per week programmed into their job plans for supporting professional activities including clinical governance.

Potential clinical governance contracts

Such an agreement might cover a number of areas.

◆ **Continuing education** planning reading, courses and study leave in a structured way that addresses the educational needs of the individual while ensuring that the resources are in place to meet these needs.

◆ **Audit** agreeing participation in a resourced audit programme that examines topics that are important quality indicators as well as others which may reflect the clinician's individual interests.

◆ **Training** establishing the training roles of the individual and the support that is needed for this activity.

◆ **Research** defining the role of research in the department and the extent of clinical and administrative support that is needed.

Chapter 11

Prioritisation & project management

It is not necessary to change. Survival is not mandatory.
Edwards Deming

Clinical governance is the process whereby we strive to deliver accountable, high quality and patient-focused healthcare. Before launching into a turbulent period of change in the name of clinical governance, it is vital that we take time to consider what it is that we are aiming for. In addition, those who are to be responsible for initiating change must understand what mechanisms and processes need to be used if planned changes are to be successfully implemented.

It is clear that there is a requirement on all healthcare workers to be involved in the delivery of clinical governance. This statement is easily made, but it hides the fact that it is difficult to know where to start when there are so many areas with room for quality improvement. Furthermore, those within the NHS who are currently feeling the pressure to deliver on clinical governance already have very widespread responsibilities within the service. Effecting change in this environment can appear a nigh on impossible task.

For those who are in this position, there are two principles governing change programmes which should be borne in mind [1]:

Principles governing change programmes

◆ The starting point of any effective change process is a clearly defined problem.

◆ Successful change is easiest in small units - a department or business unit - where goals and tasks are clearly defined.

With this in mind, individuals responsible for initiating change should not worry about seeming only to tackle relatively small issues. The problems of the larger organisation cannot usually be solved in a single sweeping effort but have to be tackled incrementally.

Furthermore, it is essential to recognise that improving the quality of patient care does not require entirely new systems. A great deal of current healthcare is good. The successes of the NHS should not be forgotten in our efforts to provide service improvement. Consider a single department within an acute Trust. Clinical governance may necessitate a series of changes taking place throughout the department, but much will not require change. In most units there will be a mix of successful and failing processes. Amongst those that are failing, some faults will lie within the department itself (and are therefore rectifiable at this level), while others will be a part of the overall structure of the organisation. With the realisation that the power to effect change does not always lie locally, comes the reality that often it does. Efforts should always be concentrated on those areas where real improvements can be made, however large or small they might be.

Finally, it is essential to realise that good project management is fundamental to the role of an effective manager. Some understanding of the tools of this particular trade is useful for the clinician who is involved in generating change. The following sections describe some of the methodology used in project management.

Identification of clinical governance projects

We are all aware of deficiencies in our services, but usually this awareness takes the form of a vague discomfiture or sense of dissatisfaction. Clear definition of the problems can often be very difficult. Some issues will generate anxiety and concern out of proportion to their seriousness while other, more critical failings will go unnoticed.

When considering quality improvement it is basic that the real problems are identified. Establishing and maintaining a log of potential problems and issues is a starting point for managing the changes that are truly needed within a unit.

A problem log may be initiated by holding a departmental 'think tank' with input from all groups, from administrative assistants to doctors. Further issues may arise out of critical incidents and complaints as part of the risk management process. Following identification of problems, the log can be used to generate a list of projects aimed at providing solutions to the various problems.

Problems and projects

Examples of problems: Numerous patient complaints regarding mixed sex wards. Difficulties with maintaining staff continuing professional development.

Examples of projects: Implementing cancer management timescales. Merging a split-site department onto a single site.

Project prioritisation

Rome was not built in a day and nor will a day be long enough to solve the problems of the health service. Project prioritisation is an essential process; without it a department's efforts will be dissipated as a result of too many projects being commenced with too few resources to support them.

Project prioritisation can be conducted in a number of ways. One approach to prioritisation is to map the perceived departmental benefit of projects against their complexity. Simple but high-impact issues should be tackled first. Less important and complex topics may be ignored altogether if the effort that would be expended on them cannot be justified. Figure 1 illustrates this approach in graphical form. A simple scoring system can be

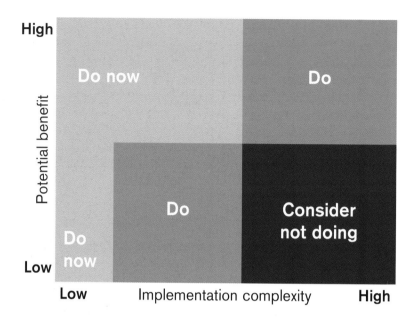

Figure 1. Project prioritisation.
(Reproduced with the kind permission of the NHS Clinical Governance Support Team).

used to stratify projects. Only those projects that can be completed within a given timescale will be started and managed through to a conclusion.

Within the NHS, as in private industry, resources are very often the limiting factor in terms of implementing change. Therefore, it is always useful to bear in mind financial, time and staffing considerations when prioritising projects. Figure 2 provides a further simple graph which can aid such decision-making. This plan focuses the mind on both the resources and time scales required for successfully taking projects forward.

Whichever way project prioritisation is achieved within a department it is important to have a balance between projects that are taken on at the same time. If possible, long-term and heavily resource-dependent projects

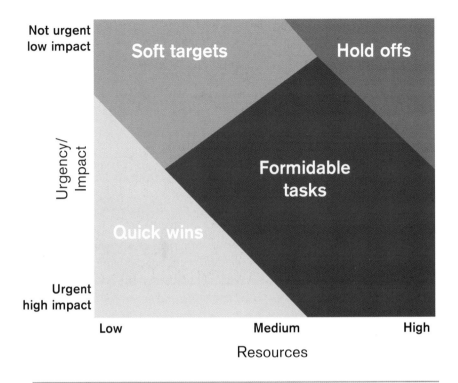

Figure 2. Project prioritisation.
(Reproduced with the kind permission of the NHS Clinical Governance Support Team).

Considerations for project prioritisation

◆ Support from colleagues, Trust Board, local General Practitioners.
◆ Presence/absence of effective clinical/managerial leaders.
◆ Dedicated project resources.
◆ Credible and experienced change leader(s).
◆ Previous history of successful project implementation.
◆ Previous history of successful change/quality improvement.
◆ Measurable outcomes.

should be run alongside short-term projects which provide immediate change. This provides those within the department with some rapid returns on their efforts and helps to maintain enthusiasm for change. Furthermore, it is vital to be realistic about the chances of carrying any project through to its conclusion before it is commenced. In addition to benefits and resources, several other factors such as support from colleagues, should be considered.

The project management process

Formal project management can itself be a cumbersome and unwieldy process. And it should be self-evident that many issues can be effectively managed without using a formal planning structure. Thus, precious time should not be squandered on planning straightforward change. However, the huge inertia within complex organisations such as the NHS must not go unrecognised. All too often, those at the top find solutions to difficulties and the problem is assumed to have been dealt with effectively; while on the clinical shop-floor the planned changes never take place. It is this phenomenon which has led to the introduction of change management tools such as RAID (see below).

Complex projects will undoubtedly require a formal project management structure. For many of those working within the NHS, the formalisation of this structure may be new and it is therefore useful to consider the process briefly.

Managing change: the RAID model

The current official teaching on the methodology of change for the NHS as a whole comes from the NHS Modernisation Agency via its clinical governance development programme [2]. The programme uses RAID (Review, Agree, Implement, Demonstrate) which can, to some degree, be applied to any defined problem (see Figure 3). The process incorporates many elements of project management and puts particular emphasis on the importance of communication and multi-disciplinary working. There

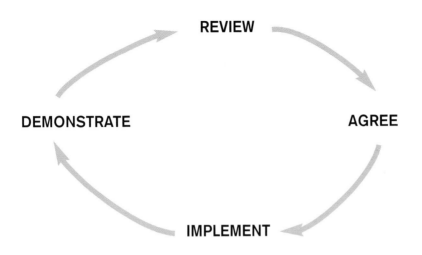

Figure 3. The RAID Model.
(Reproduced with the kind permission of the NHS Clinical Governance Support Team).

are, of course, other models that can be used such as PDSA (Plan, Do, Study, Act) which work essentially along the same lines as RAID.

Review

A multi-disciplinary review of the issues that surround the problem that is to be tackled, will allow the issue to be viewed from every angle. The aim of the review is two-fold: firstly, to define the issues and to clarify where the real difficulties lie and, secondly, to give everyone within the department a common understanding of the problem and to gain enthusiasm and commitment from them for solving it.

The review is an information-gathering exercise and a chance to heighten awareness. At this stage suggestions rather than defined solutions are required.

It is not only vital that people working within the department understand and support what is sought to be achieved, but that support for the process is also gained from those within the Trust who are ultimately responsible for clinical governance. By talking to people with a more general overview of the organisation, others may be found who have worked on the same problem, contacts may be made and pathways identified that will allow changes to be rolled out subsequently.

For the review to be successful both time and energy will be needed from members of the co-ordinating team. The review team should be multi-disciplinary and made up of individuals with the power within the organisation to effect change. There are an enormous variety of ways in which information can be gathered within a department and the aim is to involve all stakeholders.

Practical suggestions

- Workshops. These should be planned well in advance, 2 hours long, multi-disciplinary and multi-professional.
- Reviewing patient complaints.
- Assessing the number of near misses or critical incidents relating to the project area.
- Looking at the evidence for best practice - government papers, Royal College recommendations, academic articles, policies, pathways and guidelines.
- Questionnaires. Do people agree with the project's aims? What is currently done well? Where are the areas for improvement? What are the sources of personal frustration?
- One-to-one interviews. These enable the team to listen to a wide selection of frontline staff, hear their frustrations, hear their vision and their ideas for delivering improvement and encourage any willingness to actively support the initiative.
- Informal discussion. It is often said that the most useful part of any meeting occurs in the coffee room afterwards.

Through gathering this large volume of information, themes will emerge which will clarify the real problem which needs to be tackled. Hopefully a vision of how things may work in the future will also begin to emerge. From this exercise the team will be able to draw up detailed recommendations for solving the original problem and measuring success. These detailed recommendations are essentially a project proposal.

Project proposal requirements

- A project title.
- Background to the project, defining the problem to be solved.
- Overall project aims - these may extend beyond the immediate problem.
- A list of stakeholders.
- Resources required for project completion - include the source of funding, time and staff.
- A realistic project timescale - this might be easily represented with the use of a Gantt chart (Figure 4).
- The measures of success - eg. Key Performance Indicators (KPIs).
- A plan of those to be involved in the project - team members and leaders - with their roles and responsibilities.
- A communication strategy.
- A risk strategy - include each potential risk to the project, its impact, its chance of occurrence and the actions to be taken in the event of the risk being realised (Table 1).

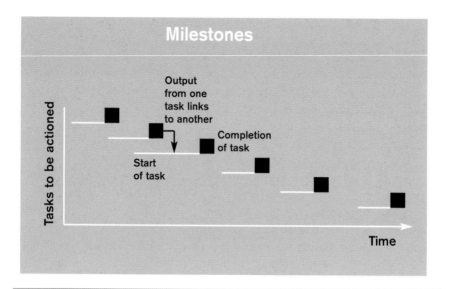

Figure 4. A Gantt chart.
(Reproduced with the kind permission of the NHS Clinical Governance Support Team).

Table 1. A risk strategy.

RISKS	LIKELIHOOD OF OCCURRENCE	IMPACT ON PROJECT	MITIGATING ACTIONS
What might get in the way of successful delivery of the project?	High/Medium/Low	High/Medium/Low	Key actions required to prevent risks happening - or to deal with them if they do arise

Agreement

The conclusions and recommendations from the review need to be agreed by all those who will be involved in taking change forward. Many of these people will have been involved in the review process itself. Others, who are not intimately involved with the workings of the department, may need to be approached in order to gain agreement for changes in policy which will affect their working environment.

If the review has been carried out effectively, writing the recommendations or project proposal should be fairly straightforward. However, agreement on the recommendations may not be so easily obtained. It is vital that all stakeholders buy in to the project before it is commenced i.e. during the review process, because without agreement the project is doomed before it has begun. Those who are funding the project will not support actions that they have not signed up to, and equally, those whose daily lives are to be affected by the project will not implement changes that they do not believe in.

Different groups and individuals will always have their own agendas when it comes to agreeing change within any organisation. It is important to recognise this from the start and to accept it. The process of agreement, if it is to be effective in marking the start of a successful change project, may well require very skilled communication and conflict resolution. The project proposal will inevitably contain elements that are not agreeable to all concerned, but which represent (hopefully) the best way forward for the department as a whole.

Remember, a project cannot move forward until everyone has bought into the recommendations.

Implementation

It may well be the case that the project that is to deliver change turns out to be multi-faceted and requires several steps to be taken in order to obtain the required improvement. There may, in effect, be a number of mini-projects which will need to be implemented. If appropriate team leaders for these mini-projects have not emerged during the review and agreement process they will need to be identified.

The implementation part of the RAID process is essentially about conducting the project/projects. Many of the skills and tools already mentioned will prove valuable throughout this process. One very important factor is that of establishing controls. If the timescale of the project was not formally mapped out within the recommendations, it is sensible to use a Gantt chart (or similar) at this stage to ensure progress can be readily monitored. Forward momentum can be ensured by checking off the pre-determined milestones. It is also important to keep an eye on the project's principal aims and to avoid diversions away from the primary task.

One further tool that is very widely used in project management is worth mentioning here: process mapping. This is a very straightforward way of looking at complex processes step by step. Single processes within healthcare can involve an enormous number of individual steps and different members of staff. An example would be providing notes for an individual patient seen in the outpatient clinic and getting them back to

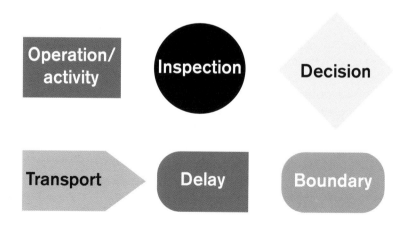

Figure 5. Process mapping shapes.
(Reproduced with the kind permission of the NHS Clinical Governance Support Team).

medical records following the generation of a clinic letter. Within such a complex process it is often difficult to find where the delays or problems lie because no single individual has an overall view of the journey of the medical notes. It is often useful therefore, to map the process in a standard format with all of those involved in the process present. This will enable everyone to recognise not only delays and difficulties, but also unnecessary steps within the system. Figure 5 shows the basic shapes for process mapping, while Figure 6 shows an example process map.

Process mapping can of course be used at any stage of the RAID process, but may well be most beneficial in aiding problem-solving during the early, planning stages.

Demonstration

The accent on being able to measure and identify beneficial change comes from an appreciation that the NHS has a long history of ineffective reform. The designers of modernisation are placing their trust in the principle that small, incremental improvements will combine into major benefits through a process of sharing best practice.

The measurement of improvement may be achieved by repeating some of the review exercises - questionnaires, interviews and so on. Furthermore the classic principles of audit can be applied to examine the effectiveness of the change process.

The introduction of the RAID methodology reflects concerns that the NHS may be stubbornly resistant to the proposed modernisation reforms in general and clinical governance-driven change in particular. The fear is that the service is fundamentally conservative (with a small 'c'). An alternative view is that many healthcare professionals are innovative and progressive by nature and that development has been slowed by the twin impediments of limited resources and organisational instability. If the latter is correct, RAID's emphasis on culture and wide involvement may be unnecessarily cumbersome; progress might be accelerated more quickly by introducing managerial and administrative support to those who already have ideas and plans in place or are willing to take on board standards of best practice that have been developed elsewhere.

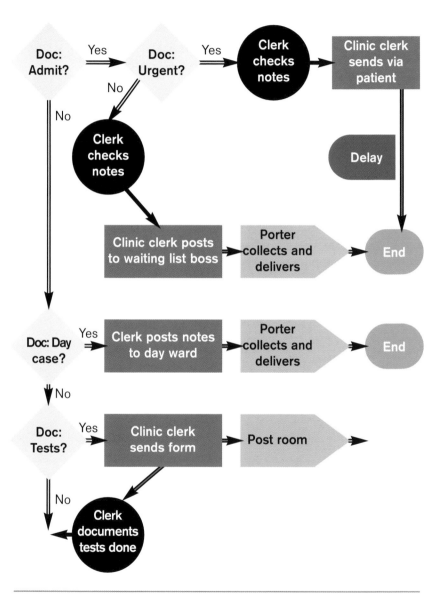

Figure 6. A process map.
(Reproduced with the kind permission of the NHS Clinical Governance Support Team).

References

1   Beer M, Eisenstat RA, Spector B. Why change programmes don't produce change. *Harvard Bus Rev* 1990 Nov-Dec; 68(6): 158-66.

2   Cullen R, Nicholls S, Halligan A. NHS Support Team. Reviewing a service - discovering the unwritten rules. *Brit J Clin Governance* 2000; 5(4):233-239.

Further reading

*   Nicholls S, Cullen R, Halligan A. Clinical governance ... after the review - what next? Agreement and implementation. *Brit J Clin Governance* 2001; 6(2).

*   Cullen R, Nicholls S, Halligan A. Measurement to demonstrate success. *Brit J Clin Governance* 2001; 6(4): 273-278.

*   Dash P. Tips On ..: Project management *BMJ* 2002; 325: S127.

PART IV

Components of clinical governance

In Part IV the time honoured strategy of divide and conquer is employed. By separating clinical governance into its, albeit overlapping, component parts, it is possible to gain an understanding of its scope and importance. Most importantly, it is possible to gain an appreciation as to how clinical governance might be able to deliver improvements in the quality of our efforts in the clinical setting.

Chapter 12
Cultural shift

*Our culture peculiarly honours the act of blaming,
which it takes as the sign of virtue and intellect.*
Lionel Trilling

Our NHS culture

The behaviour, attitudes, assumptions and values of any group or organisation make up its culture. They mix together to produce working practices - "the way things are done around here" [1]. We have a capacity to observe the culture of other groups in a critical light, while blithely displaying our own characteristics - a fault also seen when considering beauty (or the lack of it) and bad habits.

If we are born into, or nurtured within a culture, we cannot avoid developing its characteristics and playing by at least some of its rules. The vast majority of health professionals are brought up i.e. trained, within the culture of the NHS and many, being the children of health professionals, are born into it. Vocational training takes a varied group of individuals with a common interest on an educational and cultural journey. At the journey's end are people who can exercise the skills and knowledge that they have acquired but who also exhibit characteristics that demonstrate conformity with the expectations of their chosen profession and society as a whole. Being a doctor or a nurse is not just a job.

There are many strengths within NHS culture. The dedication and commitment of health professionals is not to be underestimated. Underlying the commitment of staff is also a belief in an accessible and equitable health service and the value of being part of a public service. This belief is essential to the successful implementation of clinical governance.

But the current NHS culture also has many failings. For example, overly powerful professional and managerial hierarchies, a reluctance to comment on the conduct of colleagues, excessive demands for clinical freedom and tensions between professional groups can all lead to problems.

Efforts to improve quality, as is now required, demand that we look long and hard at the positive and negative aspects of our culture. We must recognise our good and bad habits and understand their ability to help or hinder our underlying aims.

Leadership and hierarchy

The world needs leaders, but it does not follow that a leader should always be in charge. Within hospital medicine, hierarchy and the assumption of leadership are hugely evident. Hierarchy exists both within and between the professions.

In many instances, of course, hierarchy has a vital role to play. Vocational training requires lengthy apprenticeship, which would be impossible without the security of the chain of experience and command that is fundamental to both the medical and nursing professions.

There is also a knowledge hierarchy upon which referral to the secondary and tertiary care specialist services in the NHS is based. Initial patient access is to the generalist, either the community based General Practitioner (GP) or the hospital based Accident & Emergency (A&E) practitioner. Cases requiring specialist input are then referred locally, regionally, nationally or even internationally when required. In acute situations, such as cardiac arrest, health professionals are trained to rely on the hierarchies of the 'arrest team'. The function of these leaders is less traditional and stable but just as vital.

There is no problem with hierarchy in these appropriate situations where those in charge are in a qualified position of authority. However, rigid structures of hierarchy within an organisation can mean that position transcends the structure and is abused by those who hold it. When hierarchy is brought into what should be mutual territory it weakens the culture of the NHS [2].

Although the working environment and professional relationships are much more relaxed than they were a decade or so ago, every health professional will have witnessed hierarchy wielded as power. This power is wielded both within and between professional groups. The assumption that a doctor's view is inevitably superior to that of a nurse, or that a surgeon's view is superior to that of a physician, or indeed that the position of a hospital doctor is superior to that of a GP often goes unchallenged. These assumptions can be particularly limiting within a new patient-centred working environment, where multi-disciplinary teamwork is fundamental.

It is often very difficult to break down these long established barriers, especially for those in more junior positions. Many staff within their professional groups will have been trained to jump when the boss says jump, be they consultant or nursing sister. Some will even be so well trained to immediately ask "how high?". But to challenge an individual in such an established position of authority within the organisational structure can be extremely intimidating, especially for those working on short-term contracts who are relying on a good reference to obtain their next job.

In some instances, these concerns are probably well founded and a direct challenge to an individual who believes they are in charge will not be beneficial. However, there are changes that can be made at all levels of the organisation which will gradually ensure that the most appropriate individuals are involved and listened to in any given situation, rather than automatically deferring to those in a position of structural power.

Within medicine itself, there is a view that doctors do not make good leaders. Those who by default or ambition take up senior leadership roles within local or national professional organisations often find themselves lambasted most by those whom they are trying to lead. Perhaps the problem is not that doctors do not make good leaders but that doctors do not make good followers. The essential nature and culture of medical practice i.e. independence and clinical freedom, does not allow the medical cats to be herded easily [3].

Practical suggestions

- Establish multi-disciplinary meetings as an expected norm. There are many opportunities for inter-professional learning and debate that are currently wasted through habit and ignorance. So think whether other colleagues might benefit before you restrict a meeting to other groups eg. audit and critical event meetings.
- The use of evidence-based medicine encourages us all to challenge our own practice and those of others, and to seek updated information. Evidence-based information is now widely available and is no longer locked in the heads of our more experienced or senior colleagues.
- Allow juniors to take responsibility and have a leadership role for some aspect of departmental activity. This may both reduce workload for more senior members and give juniors more confidence.
- Be sympathetic to those with medical leadership roles - seek to influence rather than criticise them.
- Explore your own leadership strengths and weaknesses with a mentor.

Professional tribalism

So far we have talked about culture within the NHS as though all those who work within the organisation shared it. Of course, things are never this simple. Within any organisation, despite having a common understanding of "the way things are done around here", there are inevitable sub-groups and thus sub-cultures. Within the health service, the cultures of nursing, medicine and management are so distinct and closely-knit as to be tribal.

It is worth understanding some of the reasons behind these NHS sub-cultures. For doctors and nurses the cultural initiation begins early. During training, there is often a geographical barrier between nursing and medical students and the outside world. They are often housed in hospitals and are frequently educated in isolation from students studying other subjects. They therefore form a natural protective club.

The realities of a career within the health service also exposes those within it to situations experienced much less by the general population. Thus we see a great 'vox pop' desire for hospital soap operas and dramas on the big and small screen.

It is important that nurses and doctors find ways of coping early with issues such as grief, death and mental illness. Once qualified, the realities of working within an over-stretched health service, whilst maintaining support for patients and families, requires healthcare staff to gain strength from behind the scenes. The individual professional cultures that bond them, give a sense of mutual support, a set of common goals and understanding and a strong sense of belonging to those within.

In the face of these many strong professional sub-cultures, managers themselves have developed their own sub-cultures, frequently changing to meet the political mood of the time. We have all witnessed the private sector suited brigades of managers of the early NHS reforms. These have now been replaced with a breed of new public sector managers, whose strengths lie more in political astuteness, avoiding outlying positions in league tables and collaborative working than in any particular dress sense.

Like hierarchy, tribalism has positive aspects enabling those working within the NHS to do so with humour and generosity. But there is also a downside to tribal cultures. The close-knit atmosphere instils such a strong sense of common purpose that it can blind individuals to the purpose of others. This can mean that doctors, nurses and managers vigorously defend their own corner believing that other groups do not understand the issues or do not have the same aims. Clinical governance, in its aims towards an integrated, quality service for patients, demands that different groups of health professionals work together in teams. This is not possible if groups of professionals are placing the interests of their professional tribes before that of the patient that they are caring for.

> **Practical suggestions**
>
> - Common understanding can be gained by joint training and education. Although difficult in undergraduate training, there is no reason why barriers can not be broken down within the workplace.
> - Personally champion the need for multi-disciplinary teams and working.
> - When writing new protocols and guidelines, always try to do this from a multi-disciplinary perspective.
> - If you find yourself in a negotiation situation, or real conflict, always put yourself in the other person's shoes to understand their perspective.
> - Always try for win-win, never for win-lose.
> - As part of your personal/professional development plan, consider shadowing a colleague from another discipline (eg. nursing/management) for a short while.

Communicating with patients

The General Medical Council (GMC), in their guidance *Good Medical Practice*, spell out the duties of a doctor (see page 88). It is evident that good communication skills are a fundamental requirement for these duties.

There are, however, two major stumbling blocks in terms of analysing patient - professional communication. The first is the problem of defining quality, as already acknowledged. Arising from this is the second problem, that of agreeing what are the important quality issues to be addressed as a priority. Most health professionals, when asked to define a quality service, would put emphasis on an accurate and expedient diagnosis, technical excellence and a successful clinical outcome. Patients on the other hand will weight their list differently.

The duties of a doctor registered with the GMC are:

- make the care of your patient your first concern;
- treat every patient politely and considerately;
- respect patients' dignity and privacy;
- listen to patients and respect their views;
- give patients information in a way that they can understand;
- respect the rights of the patient to be fully involved in decisions about their care;
- keep your professional knowledge and skills up to date;
- recognise the limits of your professional competence;
- be honest and trustworthy;
- respect and protect confidential information;
- make sure that your personal beliefs do not prejudice your patients' care;
- act quickly to protect patients from risk if you have good reason to believe that you or a colleague may not be fit to practice;
- avoid abusing your position as a doctor; and
- work with colleagues in the ways that best serve patients' interests.

Based on 12 years of multi-national research, and more than 450,000 patient interviews, the Picker Institute has identified eight "dimensions of care" which reflect a patient's most important concerns (see facing page) [4].

The importance of communication is further confirmed when reading annual reports and case studies from any of the medical indemnity organisations and the NHS Ombudsman. A 1997 survey of senior NHS

A patient's greatest concerns in clinical care

◆ Respecting a patient's values, preferences and expressed needs.

◆ Access to care.

◆ Emotional support.

◆ Information, communication and education.

◆ Co-ordination of care.

◆ Physical comfort.

◆ Involvement of family and friends.

◆ Continuity and transition.

Practical suggestions

● Review recent hospital/departmental complaints to see how many relate to communication issues rather than more technical problems.

● Review or audit how well you and your team relate to patients in terms of verbal and written communication.

● Experiment with enhancing communication skills through using video consultations as used effectively within general practice training.

● Invite an experienced GP tutor to talk to your staff on how communication skills are developed in primary care.

● Involve a patient/lay person or a colleague from your Trust's Patient Advice and Liaison Service (PALS) in your departmental clinical governance planning in relation to patient communication.

doctors and managers who had experience of dealing with poorly performing doctors, found that problems of manner, attitude and communication were more frequent issues than were problems with patient management, diagnosis or prescribing [5]. A review of any Trust's complaints cases would no doubt reveal a similar pattern.

Communicating within and between professions

Healthcare is by definition a '24-7' profession. For high quality patient care to succeed it is vital that communication is good between and within the different professional groups that might be involved in the care of a single patient. The situation in an average hospital, however, does not always lend itself to ready communication between staff.

Doctors can have daily responsibility for up to 50 patients on different wards within a hospital at any one time. Additionally, on-call doctors are usually responsible for some patients whom they have never met or dealt with. We have experienced nurses having to deal with up to 15 different teams of doctors, of all specialities, doing ward-rounds on a single ward. Managers are responsible for elements of care for patients they often have never previously met, for example when dealing with complaints.

It is very easy to understand why communication is difficult in such a varied and busy service when the condition of any single patient may change minute by minute. We know that the most important issues for patients are related to communication, not just directly from staff, but between staff to enable a smooth transition for the patient through the service. This is fundamental to a quality patient service, and moreover, it is something that health professionals can do something about.

It is all too easy to stereotype members of multi-disciplinary teams into their various professional roles. Whilst this may be true as a sweeping generalisation, within each individual team/department there will be a spread of different personality types also interacting with each other. Team dynamics are likely to be affected as much by these as they are by the various team professional roles. Work to develop teams (particularly those that are dysfunctional) needs to focus on roles played by personalities in teams as well as professional boundaries [6].

Practical suggestions

- Promote the concept of the separate medical and nursing notes being part of a single 'whole patient' record by having both used during ward rounds.
- Encourage other disciplines to write relevant information in patient notes eg. dieticians, pharmacists.
- Where possible, try and avoid the use of locally accepted acronyms in notes - they can be difficult for locums to make sense of and can be misunderstood.
- Try not to go on a ward round alone. If you must, always write in the patients' notes, especially if there are specific plans for an individual patient - the on call team won't automatically know what your intended management is.
- Provisional reports should always be entered in the patient's notes as final reports may take days to arrive.
- Consider dictating your ward round notes so that a legible typed entry appears in the notes.
- Highlight diagnoses clearly to help medical coders and those writing discharge summaries.

Clinical freedom

Historically, doctors have had ultimate clinical responsibility for their patients. They have not only made direct clinical decisions related to patient care, but have also been in management positions whereby they were able to direct departmental and hospital resources. This gave individual doctors a large degree of freedom in terms of the care that their patients received; this was especially true for clinicians who were in powerful positions within the organisation.

As health professionals, doctors individually no longer have such strong influence over the care that their patients receive, either directly through clinical decision-making, or indirectly through resource distribution.

Management structures have changed enormously over the past 20 years limiting the medical influence on resource planning. In addition, the introduction of evidence-based medicine, together with increased access to international opinion has meant that doctors have much less individual choice over the care that their patients receive. It is no longer acceptable practice to continue with any technique or therapy against the tide of scientifically proven opinion.

Yet, there are those who still lay strong claim to clinical freedom. At face value it is reassuring for patients that the doctor is on their side and puts their interests first. But there remains the danger that overly-strong adherence to an individual medical point of view leaves no room for debate on the part of the patient or other professionals involved in the care process. In this situation, the specialist medical opinion is merely code for "this doctor knows best". As professional members of multi-disciplinary teams such strong stances may, at times, be counterproductive and may not always serve the best interests of the patient.

There is no longer room for excessive degrees of autonomy in large organisations where resources are limited and there are requirements to meet many different agreed standards.

Practical suggestions

- Think about resources - does the benefit of the technique/drug given to the individual outweigh the benefits of a cheaper alternative for more patients. If you were in the patient's shoes and having to pay privately without insurance cover, would you still advocate this line of action?
- Think about evidence - are you just throwing the weight of your experience around?

The blame culture

The NHS is not alone in nurturing a culture of blame over the years. A brief look at the national news on any given day will provide a multitude of stories demanding that individuals and organisations be held to account for their actions. In the world of politics mistakes often require a scapegoat too. In healthcare, there are increasing numbers of public scandals in which the public and media bay for professional blood.

In our modern society we are taught to expect excellence as a right in all aspects of life. It is not surprising, therefore, that we should want to blame someone if things do not happen as promised. The flip side of this intolerance is the effect that it has within organisations. There is huge fear within the health service of public recrimination. Health professionals do not see any room for mistakes and the culture of blame outside the organisation is naturally reflected within its walls.

But the effects of this long-standing blame culture within the NHS are far reaching. It drives under-reporting of critical incidents and fosters friction between individuals. This limits the capacity of the organisation to learn from mistakes. As a result the culture of blame is a major barrier to improving quality patient care. It is clear that reversing the tendency to look to place blame is critical if we are to advance real quality improvement in the NHS through clinical governance. The ongoing work by the Chief Medical Officer, Sir Liam Donaldson, to review the NHS Clinical Negligence Scheme could be a turning point in this respect.

A further insidious effect of a culture of fault and blame has enormous potential for harm: the development of an overly self-critical approach to medical practice. It is almost certainly the case that previous generations of clinicians were generally afforded a more supportive working environment; many clinical problems did not have solutions and to be seen to have tried one's best was often regarded as sufficient. In contrast, there is now every opportunity for adverse outcomes to be ruthlessly analysed so that lessons may be learned - but at a significant cost to self-confidence and esteem. For some practitioners, this pressure results in deteriorating clinical performance as responsibilities and decision-making become an increasing burden.

There is an essential balance that must be struck by anyone who works in healthcare. It is probably healthy to feel partly responsible for a patient's poor clinical outcome and, from time to time, to experience a few disturbed nights' sleep as events turn over in one's mind. But clinical sanity and performance depends on the ability to turn away from such reflections and concerns and to move on. Beneficial cultural shift will involve developing a means of learning from mistakes while recognising the potential costs of such knowledge.

Practical suggestions

● Respond positively rather than defensively to critical incident reporting.
● Promote anonymous open discussion of complications as well as complaints within the department.
● Lead by example within the department and discuss critical incidents involving yourself.

References

1   The Culture of the NHS. Chapter 22. The Bristol Royal Infirmary Inquiry. www.bristol-inquiry.org.uk/final_report.

2   Ibid.

3   Egger E. Like herding cats, herd physicians by making them want to come. [Congresses] *Healthcare Strategic Management* 2000; 18(7):18-9.

4   Nicholls S, Cullen R, O'Neill S, Halligan A. Clinical Governance: its origins and its foundations. *Clinical Performance and Quality Health Care* 2002; 8(3): 172-8.

5   Hutchinson A, Williams M, Meadows K, Barbour RS, Jones R. Perceptions of good medical practice in the NHS: a survey of senior health professionals. *Quality in Health Care* 1999; 8: 213-218.

6   Belbin RM. Building effective management teams. *Journal of General Management* 1976; 3(3): 23-9.

Further reading

• NHS Ombudsman (Health Service Commissioner). www.ombudsman.org.uk/hse/index.html.
• Read case summaries of medical indemnity organisations' annual reports.
• Learning from Bristol: report of the public inquiry into children's heart surgery at the Bristol Royal Infirmary 1984-1995. The Stationery Office, Norwich, 2001. (especially the culture of public service section: www.bristol-inquiry.org.uk/final_report/report/sec2chap22_9.htm).
• Hampton JR. The end of clinical freedom. *BMJ* 1983; 287: 1237-1238.
• Klein R. *The politics of the National Health Service*. Longman, London, 1983.

Chapter 13

Risk management

How wonderful it is that nobody need wait a single
moment before starting to improve the world.
Anne Frank

It is notoriously difficult to communicate the concepts of chance and risk and yet a mature appreciation of medical interventions can only be achieved when meaning has been given to such ideas. We work in daily contact with the scales that weigh risk and benefit and yet healthcare workers have not always been effective in their management of risk. Clinical governance puts risk management centre stage and consequently poses the question: how do we deal more effectively with the dangers that are inherent in medical practice? This is a much wider and more open arena than that provided historically by the confines of medical negligence-avoidance.

In this chapter we examine the context of risk management in clinical governance, what we mean by risk, error and failure, and define the components of good risk management. Finally we explore some of the more topical and challenging practical aspects of risk management for healthcare professionals in today's NHS.

Context of risk management

Recognising a need

Risk management is still a relatively new concept in healthcare. Prior to the mid 1980s most risk management specialists had concentrated their efforts and expertise on much more conspicuous catastrophes. Accidents occurring in hazardous industries such as air-travel, shipping, nuclear power and chemical processing can have a devastating and widespread impact. The enormous cost of such individual accidents, in both human life and environmental damage, together with the surrounding public and political concern, make them obvious targets for risk management input. In contrast, accidents occurring within healthcare (other than those involving population health programmes such as cancer screening) tend to affect individual patients and to occur in a variety of institutions spread across the country. Thus, the true impact of adverse events in medicine and the need for risk management in health was historically less obvious than in some other industries.

The introduction of risk management into healthcare was driven in part, by the realisation that medicine did have its own disasters such as the thalidomide crisis. But, perhaps the strongest driver was the escalation in medical litigation with its associated damage to healthcare budgets and professional reputations. As the public began to demand financial recompense for medical accidents, the NHS recognised the need for a preventative response. But despite its original function as a defence against weighty compensation payments, risk management rapidly acquired its own impetus, as the true cost of medical accidents became apparent. The financial burden of negligence claims will always be far outweighed by the costs of hospitalisation and sickness benefits that arise from adverse events within healthcare. The cost in terms of individual suffering could not be ignored, but quality improvements are most easily achieved if the financial impact allows a win-win result.

Thus, risk management was introduced to healthcare. As the positive influence of risk management has become recognised so has the need for collaboration with specialists in risk analysis. If the aim of limiting the numbers and impact of medical accidents is to be achieved, some understanding of the causes of errors has to be grasped. Much has also to be learned about the design of strategies that most effectively avoid or limit such mistakes.

The impact of clinical governance

Initially, it was those working in anaesthetics and intensive care who were targeted for risk management consideration. These jobs were thought to have much in common with jobs in other industries where risk management strategies had been developed over many years and were highly sophisticated. Gradually, the need to extend risk management throughout the whole field of healthcare activity has become clear.

Despite such recognition, healthcare workers have, in general, not been well informed regarding the wider picture of medical risk. Additionally, there remain notable contradictions in the practice of medicine at the present time. Some medical risks, such as the prevention of infection in joint replacement surgery, are tackled with vigour and at considerable cost. Such action is undoubtedly correct despite the low probability of occurrence, when the outcome of such an adverse event for the individual patient is disastrous. On the other hand, there is a tendency for us to accept some much more frequently occurring and quite significant risks, when they can be categorised as administrative. For example, it is frequently accepted that patients with serious conditions can get "lost in the system" as a result of an inability to track people along investigation and treatment pathways.

With the introduction of clinical governance, risk management in healthcare has moved to centre stage. Whilst NHS Trust Boards for many years have had to focus on managing risk in its widest sense as part of good corporate governance and controls assurance, clinical governance now poses the question: how do we more effectively deal with all of the dangers that are inherent within clinical practice itself? Substantial quality improvement will only be achieved by reducing the occurrence of all categories of risk.

With the creation of the new National Patient Safety Agency (NPSA) we now see strong evidence that the government sees risk management as a central component of good clinical governance. The NPSA aims to encourage open reporting of adverse events and near misses in healthcare and to learn from these across all healthcare organisations.

Understanding risk

Fundamental to an understanding of risk is an appreciation of the enormous contribution humans make to medical accidents and adverse events. Figures for the human error component of accidents in environments such as medicine have been shown to be as high as 90%[1]. Much research has been undertaken in this area and the all-important human contribution to risk can now be categorised.

Firstly, errors can be distinguished from violations. Errors are defined as the failure of an action to produce the desired result. In comparison, violations are usually deliberate and entail cutting corners or ignoring rules and regulations. Violations generally relate to poor motivation or low morale. Errors arise either from straightforward lapses, where the task is simply not performed correctly, or in the form of mistakes, where the execution of the task or plan is performed correctly but the plan itself was flawed (Figure 1).

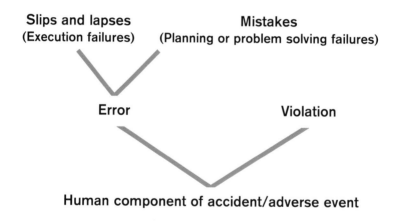

Slips and lapses
(Execution failures)

Mistakes
(Planning or problem solving failures)

Error

Violation

Human component of accident/adverse event

Figure 1. The human component of accidents and adverse events.

Secondly, in understanding the human contribution to adverse events it is important to draw a distinction between active and latent failures. Active failures are the unsafe acts that occur most proximally to the adverse event, performed by the individuals at the point of delivery of care. These are failures by those on the shop-floor that can directly harm the individual patient. In contrast, latent failures are created within the organisational structure of the healthcare system and may lie dormant for a very long time. Latent failures will become evident only when they combine with local factors to produce an adverse event.

Reducing the risk of drug errors

Drug administration errors are a good example of an area where risk management is essential. Throughout the health service drug errors are exceedingly common and are also potentially very serious. Reducing the chance of such errors occurring involves looking at issues from prescription to drug delivery.

Each individual step in the drug administration process has the potential for an active or latent adverse event.

◆ Prescription writing.
◆ Drug labelling.
◆ Drug delivery to the site of administration.
◆ Staff training.
◆ The actions of the individual who identifies the patient and administers the drug.
◆ The local environment at the time of drug administration.

At an organisational level, drug errors should be monitored and reviewed as a group of errors to look for systematic problems. For the individual department, review of a single error may throw up lessons which are specific to the particular situation, such as nurses being repeatedly interrupted during drug rounds; the solution for which may be to adjust the timing of the drug round.

Active failures

A Late one Saturday night a 51 year old man presents to a busy Accident & Emergency department complaining of chest pain following a heavy meal. His ECG is recorded by the SHO (who is alone in the department) as showing no abnormalities. Cardiac enzymes are just within normal limits. A diagnosis of gastritis is given and he is discharged home. The following day he collapses and dies. On review, the ECG shows clear ischaemic changes.

B A 73 year old woman with known superficial bladder cancer fails to respond to a letter asking her to attend for a check cystoscopy. Her name is subsequently removed from the waiting list by administrative staff. Eleven months later she sees her GP complaining of frank haematuria and is re-referred to the Urology department where an urgent cystoscopy is arranged for her. This reveals recurrent bladder cancer which is now invasive.

C Following emergency surgery for a spinal abscess a 37 year old man is transferred to a medical ward where he is nursed on a standard mattress. He has reduced mobility associated with his slowly resolving neuropathy and rapidly develops a deep sacral pressure sore.

D A 34 year old woman attends the Day Surgery Unit for varicose vein surgery. Whilst in the anaesthetic room the anaesthetist requests 1ml of 1% lignocaine for injection in order to ease the discomfort of the anaesthetic drug propofol. Her assistant hands her 1ml of adrenaline instead. The anaesthetist checks the vial and notices the problem, thus averting a serious drug administration error.

Latent failures

A Departments regularly rely on inexperienced staff to cover unsociable duty hours. Junior staff in this situation may feel pressured by both time and the absence of a sufficient support mechanism to make clinical decisions beyond their experience.

B A lack of inherent clinical checks within a waiting list validation exercise.

C Bed shortages and bed sharing between specialties mean that patients are often cared for on wards where the staff are unfamiliar with the diagnoses and special requirements of patients.

D Drug vials are designed to be as cheap as possible and therefore many very different drugs are stored in exactly the same kind of vials.

Adverse events or accidents in complex organisations such as healthcare are generally the consequence of a series of failures. First, there are the organisational or latent failures in terms of the design, planning and forecasting, which create the structured environment in which we work. Second, there are contributory or triggering factors, such as under-staffing and high workload, which increase the probability of failures actually occurring through subsequent human errors and violations. On the whole, catastrophes occur only when such a series of failures occurs together.

This type of analysis leads to a realisation that reductions in the numbers of adverse events will occur as a result of improving the knowledge, motivation and effectiveness of the whole team of individuals who are involved in the delivery of care. Particularly important is the issue of ensuring good communications. The alternative approach of directing energy at investigating events and designing local protocols to try to prevent recurrences of the incident is likely to be relatively ineffective if the team involved remains poorly trained and demotivated. An over-emphasis on individual incidents, finding fault and blame allocation is to be avoided. It may give short-term gratification to those who sit in judgement but it will do little to protect future patients. The goal that should be sought is the creation of a motivated team who understand their roles, are well trained and, crucially, communicate well at all levels.

Components of risk management

Identifying Risk

The starting point for the process of risk management has to be risk identification. And in turn, the starting point for risk identification is for all those working within the NHS to have a naturally risk-aware approach. The significance and importance of individual actions and responsibilities in terms of identifying risk should not be underestimated or ignored.

In devastating circumstances, when a patient has suffered significant injury or death, risk identification may be relatively straightforward. In such instances questions will naturally be asked and a significant effort put into understanding and reporting the chain of events leading to such a significant adverse event. But in a different situation, where no actual injury or damage has occurred, or it has been narrowly avoided, it is more difficult to identify risk.

The problems with good risk management in these 'near-miss' situations are two-fold. First, staff who realise that they have narrowly escaped being involved in a significant adverse incident will not necessarily report it. Many staff will breathe a sigh of relief and make a mental note to themselves to not make the same mistake again. Those witnessing such an incident often react in a similar way. The resistance to reporting any such incident often arises from a fear of being blamed by others for such a mistake, or indeed simply of appearing fallible in front of colleagues. In addition, staff may not know how or to whom to report such a risk. Or they may simply be too busy to find and complete the incident notification document.

The second problem is that staff involved in high-risk events simply may not recognise them as such. If staff are unaware of significant risks or adverse incidents around them, any risk management process will inevitably be poor. For example, it is evident that seeing patients without the appropriate medical notes is a high-risk activity, especially when undertaking any procedure upon a patient or changing medical management. However, members of staff may not necessarily recognise this risk, or may not feel empowered within the system to refuse to see a patient or to cancel a procedure. Therefore, it is vital that all departmental staff understand what sort of activities are high risk and why they should be reported, and that they learn to recognise them. In addition, it is equally important that the reporting process for risks and adverse events is made simple and user friendly.

One way of formalising this approach is for a clinical department to maintain a risk register. The register can be updated as and when new risks are identified, or previously identified difficulties are eliminated. Ideally, as described above, risks are detected by the realisation that there is a weakness which might lead to a problem rather than risks always being identified because an adverse event has actually occurred. Of course, critical incident reports also have to be entered into the registration process. Consideration should be given to logging departmental incidents not only by using a standard incident report form but also by e-mail or other rapid and low-effort system in order to capture more data. The register should be regularly reviewed and updated at clinical governance meetings. The NPSA are working to develop a standardised electronic reporting form for use throughout the NHS for near miss and actual incidents.

Having identified potential problems, it is necessary to develop a strategy to deal with the issues; this requires prioritisation based on an analysis of the registered risks. It is not sensible, or necessary, for every department to design and manage a unique risk register. Examples of good practice or effective modification of a usual system are worth recording and reviewing. It will be far more useful in the long run for departments to have a benchmark, against which to compare themselves. The Clinical Negligence Scheme for Trusts and the NPSA may provide such a starting point.

The Clinical Negligence Scheme for Trusts (CNST) was established in 1995 in order to provide insurance against clinical negligence claims. Part of the scheme's role is to reduce or contain the level of such claims. One approach to this has been to introduce standards which can be used as a template for reviewing risk management mechanisms in an organisation. However, the standards have relatively little relevance to the individual who is working on the 'shop floor'; the process is essentially a top down one. On the other hand, the standards do serve to emphasise the importance of reporting and monitoring clinical incidents, maintaining robust procedures for providing information and obtaining consent, and the crucial role of good medical records and effective medical records administration.

A further source of information and ideas as to where areas of risk might lie is the NPSA. This organisation aims to identify errors and adverse events (largely using an anonymous approach), with a view to disseminating information that will allow risk avoidance elsewhere in the NHS. It is hoped that this systematic, national approach to problems will produce mechanisms which will alter current NHS systems and practice in the direction of enhanced patient safety.

Practical suggestions

- Champion a no blame culture within both clinical teams and departments.
- Educate staff regarding risk registration and reporting.
- Maintain a departmental risk register.
- Link any new risk reporting mechanism to ongoing practices within the Trust.
- Make sure risk reporting mechanisms are easy to use.
- Encourage risk reporting by thanking those who report risks/adverse events.
- Review the departmental risk register regularly.

Risk analysis techniques

It can be argued that risk identification is a process which is now becoming established, if not refined, within the NHS. Unfortunately the knowledge that adverse events occur is not, in itself, protective. A process of analysis must be followed if a safer health environment is to be achieved.

There is, unfortunately, an abundance of raw material produced by adverse incidents and near misses that might be examined; a typical hospital Trust will log several thousand clinical incidents and complaints per year; an individual department will therefore have dozens of potential areas for consideration. Thus, prioritisation is essential if efforts are going to be rewarded with real risk reductions.

Once a decision has been made to address a particular topic, an analysis has to be undertaken that allows a solution to be designed which will reduce future risk. In the past, the culture of the NHS has made such analysis difficult. But fortunately, the philosophy behind risk analysis is now becoming more widely accepted within the health service and the days when a clinician could carry an argument using the 'shroud-waving' approach are now gone. A structured approach to risk-evaluation is therefore valuable as an aid to clarify thinking and to enable objective risk prioritisation.

The risk analysis process can be carried out at a highly sophisticated level, as demonstrated very publicly within a number of industries. For example, within the transport sector, investment in rail safety technology is guided by calculations of the number of pounds spent per life saved. In medicine, similar techniques can be used to assess the balance between risk and benefit of a treatment intervention. Carotid endarterectomy for stroke prophylaxis is an example where such an approach has allowed evaluation of the efficacy of the procedure.

Productive risk analysis must cover the issues of both probability and severity. In addition, analysis must not focus exclusively on individual staff members but must look at the system as a whole. One widely used tool for risk analysis is a simple grid which plots risk impact against the probability of the harmful event arising (Tables 1 and 2). As with all such

Risk analysis for carotid endarterectomy

Carotid endarterectomy aims to reduce the risk of stroke and death in patients with carotid artery disease.

Large international trials have quantified risk and benefit of carotid endarterectomy in both symptomatic and asymptomatic patients [2,3]. Benefit of endarterectomy has been shown in patients with a high degree of stenosis:

Symptomatic patients with >70% stenosis:

◆ 26.5% three-year risk of stroke and death with best medical therapy.
◆ 14.9% three-year risk of stroke and death with carotid endarterectomy.

Post-operative surgical risk of stroke and death = 7%
7 operations are required to prevent 1 stroke

Asymptomatic patients with >60% stenosis:

◆ 11% five-year risk of stroke and death with best medical therapy.
◆ 5.1% five-year risk of stroke and death with carotid endarterectomy.

Post-operative surgical risk of stroke and death = 2.3%
50 operations are required to prevent 1 disabling stroke

Thus there is Grade A evidence that carotid endarterectomy reduces the risk of stroke and death in patients with both symptomatic and asymptomatic carotid artery disease.

techniques, it is important to remain aware of the limitations of the analysis and to question both the validity and accuracy of the assumptions that are used to construct the grid.

Table 1. Incident risk level estimator risk rating chart [4].
(Reproduced with the kind permission of BMJ Books. Secker-Walker J, Taylor-Adams S. Clinical Incident Reporting. In: Clinical Risk Management: Enhancing Patient Safety, 2nd Ed. Vincent C (Ed). BMJ Books, London, 2001: 431).

| | FREQUENCY | | | |
	VERY LIKELY 4	LIKELY 3	LESS LIKELY 2	UNLIKELY 1
Very severe 4	16	12	8	4
Serious 3	12	9	6	3
Less serious 2	8	6	4	2
Not serious 1	4	3	2	1

(SEVERITY on vertical axis)

Table 2. Risk rating calculation [4].
(Reproduced with the kind permission of BMJ Books. Secker-Walker J, Taylor-Adams S. Clinical Incident Reporting. In: Clinical Risk Management: Enhancing Patient Safety, 2nd Ed. Vincent C (Ed). BMJ Books, London, 2001: 431).

Using the Incident Risk Level Estimator, consider both the expected frequency of the risk and the potential outcome. The calculated risk rating number can then be used to determine the action that is required:

Potential frequency x Potential Severity = Risk Rating Number (RRN)

RRN	Situation	Action
12-16	Intolerable, unacceptable	Stop activity
6-9	Substantial, very high risk	
3-4	Moderate, significant risk	
1-2	Tolerable, low risk	

Vincent and colleagues have developed a more comprehensive structure for investigating and analysing serious incidents and problems. This approach examines specific events and actions within the immediate and wider context. Crucially, the protocol covers the investigation process as well as providing an analysis structure. The end product of the process is the production of a report with recommendations and suggested time-scales for each suggested action. The report includes positive findings of good practice (the protocol is available from the Association of Litigation and Risk Management, Royal Society of Medicine).

Practical suggestions

- Decide how risk analysis is to be performed prior to expending energy on extensive risk identification and investigation.
- Use simple and recognised techniques for risk analysis.
- If undertaking departmental risk analysis, link in to current Trust techniques.

Reducing and eliminating risk

Once risks or adverse events have been reported, and fault identified through appropriate analysis, preventative action is required. Currently, huge efforts are being made to contain risk throughout the NHS.

Examples of NHS risk reduction programmes

- Estates management - maintenance of the safe working environment.
- Fire education programmes.
- Lifting and handling policies.
- Radiation protection.
- Patient identification procedures.
- Swab counts in the operating theatre.
- Hand washing policies.
- Yellow form reporting scheme for medicine-related adverse events.

One of the first responsibilities of the individual is to ensure that there is knowledge of, and compliance with, the (usually numerous) policies that relate to such clinical and non-clinical risks. Knowledge of these local guidelines and policies will undoubtedly go a long way towards departmental risk containment. However, it is all too often assumed that newcomers to a department will automatically have taken local policies on board in the absence of adequate guidance. Therefore it is imperative that all staff should be informed of, or better still shown, all policies relevant to their work. Leading by example in practising and encouraging others to engage in good practice is a powerful first step towards risk-reduction.

Knowledge regarding risk will only be used effectively to reduce adverse events if individuals communicate with those around them. As already acknowledged in Chapter 12, modern medicine is a 24-hour a day, seven days a week enterprise; in order to manage any patient without mistakes being made, people need to talk to each other. Such open and clear lines of communication must apply to all members of the clinical team: medical, nursing and administrative. For example, advice must be sought, and readily given, where a junior member of the team is working beyond their level of expertise. But it is equally important for the more senior individuals to be clear in giving instructions and identifying their clinical management plans. Examples of this are the clear documentation of post-operative instructions and ensuring that the management plan for a patient who has been admitted as an emergency is written in the medical notes during the post-take ward round.

Modern medical practice, apart from being continuous, is extraordinarily complex. Large numbers of individuals work in an interrelated manner on complex tasks that often fall outside routine systems. Thus, it is no wonder that the era of drawing in managers from industry in order to improve the running of the health service was short-lived. There is often no comparison between the complexities of the NHS and those of most industries. However, some areas of patient care can be given the production line treatment, by introducing care based on protocols and guidelines. Such protocols and guidelines are targeted towards designated groups of patients with specific symptoms, rather than the blanket approach to patient care which is provided by the national risk reduction programmes mentioned above. Care pathways offer the most structured form of this approach.

The introduction of National Service Frameworks (NSFs) in the NHS is one clear attempt to create a national benchmark for service development. By clarifying national service and care standards it is hoped to reduce risk of variation in care in important healthcare areas such as coronary heart disease, mental health and diabetes.

But, guideline use is not foolproof. Prior to introducing any new departmental guidelines it is important to consider whether the specific guidelines chosen are really appropriate and helpful, and also when and how they are to be reviewed.

Considerations for the introduction of guidelines

◆ What areas of practice might benefit most from guidelines?

◆ Is there a validated national protocol available?

◆ Is a selected guideline in date and how long is it likely to remain valid?

◆ How is the guideline to be disseminated?

◆ Is it appropriate and if so, how is its implementation and impact to be audited?

It is also fundamental when designing new guidelines within a department to ensure that they really are departmental and not written by individual enthusiasts in contradiction to the practices of those around them. When used as a tool to guide juniors to the differing preferences of individual consultants, guidelines can cause confusion and potentially even increase risk. The important educational impact of guidelines can be enhanced by using them as a starting point for topic discussions in departmental clinical meetings.

Where risks are apparent to the clinician but their resolution is beyond local control, it is incumbent upon the individual to identify the risk to the organisation's management. Highlighting such risks should usually be done through the Risk Management Committee and/or the clinical governance lead within your department. Presenting an argument regarding clear local risks with supporting analysis and quantification will increase the likelihood of appropriate action being taken. This responsibility is enshrined in the General Medical Council's (GMC) standards laid out in *Good Medical Practice* [5]. The significance of tackling the latent failures in an organisation is great if one accepts that preventable errors tend to occur as a result of a task being performed in an inherently flawed system.

Practical suggestions

● Make sure you have individual knowledge of Trust risk reduction programmes.
● Lead by example in following your Trust's risk reduction policy.
● Use both Trust policy and local guidelines as educational tools within departmental clinical governance meetings.
● Don't rashly introduce local protocols and guidelines - they need to be regularly updated and should be truly departmental.

Risk management in practice

We now look at three areas of risk management in practice. The issues of written and verbal communication, patient consent, and dealing with under-performance in colleagues involve some of the most challenging changes to our professional practice being driven by clinical governance.

Communication and documentation

Communication skills now receive justifiable attention in the medical and nursing training curricula. However, relatively few consultant and senior nursing staff will have had any formal training in this area and, for some, it shows! In a number of chapters already we have emphasised that communication for healthcare staff has to be efficient at many levels: with the patient, within the immediate clinical team, with other clinical units, with those in the management structure and with others such as lawyers and the media. Communication comprises not only the all-important verbal skills that are essential to clinical practice, but also many forms of written communication. It is essential to remember that improving skills is a practical proposition at every stage of seniority and in whatever capacity you work.

Good verbal communication skills are absolutely essential for all NHS staff, but perhaps especially for those with direct patient contact. Having a pleasant bedside manner is undoubtedly important, but this is just one element of verbal communication. In terms of risk reduction, being able and willing to conduct an open, honest and frank discussion with both patients and colleagues will have a far greater effect. There is little point in being essentially friendly and nice if patients and colleagues are not fully aware of your actions and plans in relation to patient care.

Despite the importance of our verbal interactions, written communication has historically been the backbone of care within the NHS. But it now seems that we live in an age of transition in clinical record keeping. The old, trusted systems, based on paper, have been overwhelmed by the complexity of modern medicine and, in many areas, insufficient resources. All too often, case records are either missing or falling apart under the strain of bloated clinical, nursing and laboratory documentation. As this time-honoured approach fails, the new dawn of electronic record keeping seems to be tantalisingly far off. Despite these problems, there is no alternative but to accept that good quality medical records remain fundamental to patient safety and good quality medical care. So, how can staff work to overcome the limitations of current medical records systems?

Clinicians have a clear personal responsibility with regard to medical records. Standards of note keeping have been laid down by the Royal Colleges and are illustrated below. Good personal practices should be supported by an insistence that other members of the team are educated regarding the required standards and aspire to them. It is no good the consultant surgeon extolling the virtues of good record keeping if he or she does not set the appropriate example by ensuring that their operating note is filed correctly before the patient leaves the operating theatre.

Techniques that may be used to improve record management include specific notes audits where the whole team of medical, nursing and administrative staff set time aside to assess current standards. This should lead to a search for ways of improving the content of the record and the intra-departmental processes covering such things as notes availability, results filing and content of written and dictated records.

Requirements for good note-keeping

◆ Patient name, hospital number and date of birth should be documented on each sheet of the medical notes.

◆ Notes should be written chronologically.

◆ Notes should be entered with the current date and time of entry.

◆ Legible handwriting is essential where notes are not typed.

◆ Offensive or derogatory remarks regarding a patient should not be entered in the medical record.

◆ All entries should be signed along with the name and contact number of the person writing in the medical notes.

◆ Alterations should rarely be made and should be explained, signed and dated.

The use of dictated records is well established in the outpatient setting but less often applied to recording in-patient care. In this arena, standard practice has often been for the most junior doctor on the ward round to act as scribe. The result is often a résumé of the patient contact that does not record the information that the more senior doctor might feel to be important.

One way of improving this process is for a dictated note to be made regarding each patient. Some specialities have embraced this habit with obvious benefits; the pressure on secretarial time is one restraint to the generation of a typed record, but it is the case that typed ward round and operation notes are becoming increasingly popular. It is up to us all to ensure that any tendency to over-verbosity is curbed and that the dictated notes retain the characteristic of pithy efficiency.

Hospital medical records systems represent complex mini-organisations that attract attention when problems arise but otherwise run in the clinical background and receive little attention from clinical staff. Undoubtedly efficiency in such systems can decline in the face of steadily increasing demands which tend not to have been matched by appropriate investment in facilities, systems and personnel.

How can the individual influence the workings of their records department? The answer lies in efficient intra-departmental administrative practices. The avoidance of unnecessarily late clinic cancellations or alterations, returning notes promptly and not hoarding piles of notes without good cause are commonly disregarded rules. But, more importantly, we should not forget our ability to influence the general culture by personal example; an insistence on certain standards, such as correctly filed results and notes availability in out-patient clinics, will help to put in place appropriate levels of care with regards to clinical records. The flexibility of staff and a willingness to cope can conspire to allow the medical records functions to slide into a sub-standard service with the attendant risks for patients.

Consent

The process of obtaining patients' consent for treatment has rightly received much attention over recent years. However, a major driver for change has come from the threat of legal action when consent has not been seen to have been appropriately obtained. This accent on the negative has been accompanied by the supposition that United Kingdom practice will come to mirror the unwieldy consent processes that are seen in the United States. Clinical governance seeks to add a different dimension: how can the process of obtaining consent be improved in a way which ensures genuine patient understanding of and agreement to their management? Improvements in consent procedures should come as a result of several areas of change within health practice.

Mechanisms for improving consent procedures

◆ Healthcare workers will be better informed about their responsibilities in relation to consent issues.

◆ The process of gaining consent, rather than reliance on the written consent form, will be seen to be the most important.

◆ Techniques for getting information across to patients should become more effective.

◆ The public will continue to learn that they have to actively contribute to the process of making informed decisions in relation to their care.

◆ The recognition that obtaining informed consent to treatment is important will support the (at present rather gradual) shift towards a less frenetic approach to medical practice; outpatient and general practice consultations are being lengthened as the need for more detailed patient/doctor discussions are being appreciated.

Several excellent publications from the Department of Health, Royal Colleges and medical indemnity/defence organisations have set out the legal framework, ethics and practicalities of obtaining patient consent. The following paragraphs aim to pick out some themes that illustrate how this area has been affected by the clinical governance approach.

Informed consent requires information. This immediately creates a major difficulty for medical practitioners because it is well recognised that many patients have relatively poor comprehension and retention of information that is provided in standard clinical consultations. If one applies a consumerism model to healthcare then the patient might be expected to take some responsibility for this failure on the principle of *caveat emptor*. However, the fragmentation of the concept of a paternalistic health service is not that complete!

In the face of the need to offer better and more accessible information several practical measures can be taken by clinicians:

Practical suggestions

- Undertake an Internet trawl for patient information leaflets. Once good examples are located, have them customised to an in-house format and ensure that their availability is guaranteed at relevant locations.
- Refuse requests to write patient information leaflets unless you are skilled in writing for a lay audience and have back-up from people with expertise in producing such literature.
- Develop routines for sending procedure-specific information when the patient is sent admission or appointment details.
- For complex interventions, counselling from several individuals can be valuable. For example, stoma care nurses are often highly skilled in this area and will provide a different perspective to that given by the surgeon who is going to create the stoma.
- Only the simplest of procedures can be covered adequately in a single consultation. If two or more detailed discussions are needed then this must be programmed into the patient's treatment pathway. For elective surgical procedures, the increasing use of pre-admission clinics and on-the-day admissions mean that final discussions cannot effectively take place on the ward and must therefore occur in another setting. One option is to run pre-admission clinics at a time when appropriately senior medical staff are available to take consent, perhaps at the end of a ward round or during an outpatient clinic; this may have to be at the cost of fewer patients being seen in the session.
- Consider different formats for information giving such as video/audiotape/Trust website.
- Use the Patient Advice and Liaison Service (PALS) to identify good quality patient information leaflets or to seek advice on those that you are writing.

The information that a patient might reasonably expect to receive will include:

Information requirements for patients giving consent

◆ A description of their condition and the natural history of the ailment if left untreated.

◆ Details of all the standard treatment approaches, even if the treating clinician has a personal preference for one particular approach to the problem.

◆ Potential side-effects and complications of the possible treatments. The clinician is advised that they should discuss all significant risks which would affect the judgement of a reasonable patient.

◆ An indication as to the experience of the treating team and the outcomes that they believe their team delivers.

Furthermore, it is clear that current expectations are that the consent procedure will involve discussions between the patient and a professional who has sufficient experience and training to be able to reach the point where the patient is making a valid, informed judgement about their treatment. Early attempts to define whether a practitioner was capable of undertaking the consent process were not entirely logical; guidance suggested that consent should only be obtained by an individual who was capable of competently performing the procedure in question. It is now recognised that it is appropriate for a variety of individuals, including nurse specialists, to undertake the consent process - the essential requirements include adequate knowledge of the procedure, training and communication skills.

The change in emphasis that has accompanied recent reviews of the approach to consent holds the concept of joint decision-making as being important. This means that clinicians are expected to discuss all reasonable approaches to a problem. This leaves a doctor or therapist in a situation where they have to discuss alternatives to a far greater degree than was formerly the case; to fail to discuss relevant options during the consenting process is no longer acceptable. This process epitomises the shift towards patient centredness; the individual is free to choose the direction of their treatment once the clinical team has discharged its responsibility to ensure that the appropriate evidence has been made available in a form which is comprehensible to the specific patient.

One area of communication that has been highlighted is that of how the clinician is to convey the probability of an outcome occurring. The language used in such discussions is often so vague as to verge on the meaningless. For example, a risk of a particular side-effect of a drug might be described as being rare or unlikely. The use of odds or percentages is more likely to be accurately understood. For situations where a clinician is repeatedly giving the same information, preparation of a chart or table might help discussions with patients eg. when discussing risks and benefits of hormone replacement therapy.

Documentation of the consent process is vital from the defensive medico-legal perspective but can also help to structure progress through the stages of information-giving, discussion and decision-making. Specific notes should be made in cases where there is doubt about a patient's capacity to understand the issues and therefore give informed consent; specific procedures apply in such cases.

There is a distinction to be made between incapacity and occasions where a patient chooses a course that is felt to be ill advised because of their individual beliefs or values. In other circumstances, patients will ask the treating clinician to take a decision regarding medical management and will indicate that they want to receive only limited information. That is the patient's prerogative and it is sensible to clearly document that they had requested such an approach.

Under-performing colleagues

The medical profession existed in a state of high public esteem and enjoyed a largely uncritical environment over the years up to the 1980s.

Professional self-regulation was largely unquestioned and the prevailing culture was such that doctors were highly protective of each other, even to the extent of covering up for colleagues who were unfit to practice. Several forces have been gradually eroding this position, namely, changing public and media attitudes, increasing use of medical negligence litigation and a more self-critical approach by doctors and other healthcare professionals. However, the history books are likely to point to the inquiry into paediatric heart surgery in Bristol as a defining event which was to alter the approach to poor performance.

It can be argued that the medical profession, their political masters and the media have created a damaging situation that threatens to break the bond of trust between the public and their healthcare services. Media presentation of medical issues has a tendency to polarise between stories about 'top doctors' working modern medical miracles and the sensationalist reporting of medical errors.

The medico-legal context is also unhelpful. Issues are frequently judged on the basis of an idealised professional world where thoughtful clinical decisions are made by well educated, communicative clinicians (who obsessionally chronicle their every decision and action). Where is the world of overbooked clinical sessions, interruptions by 'phone and bleep and endless meetings? The danger in failing to recognise that the real clinical world plays to different rules lies in the possibility that clinicians might withdraw into a low-throughput, protectionist mode of practice which is unable to deliver an adequate service volume. Furthermore, the stresses of working in modern medicine are exacerbated by the addition of further layers of unattainable expectations; the recommendations of the Bristol inquiry itself, whilst laudable, lack in places an anchor of reality.

Unfortunately, while there is widespread agreement that things must change, a coherent new approach to performance issues has yet to become established. In 1999, the government, in a consultation paper *Supporting doctors, protecting patients*, published the framework upon which reform was to be based. This paper set the scene in relation to the establishment of standards, the professional self-regulation process and the means of detecting and dealing with defective performance.

The new National Clinical Assessment Authority (NCAA) has yet to demonstrate outcomes in terms of enhanced professional practice for those referred into it. The impact of the review of the structure and function of the General Medical Council (GMC) with greater lay power and new accountability to the new Council for the Regulation of Healthcare Professionals remains to be seen.

The publication of *Good Medical Practice* by the GMC has been extremely helpful in emphasising the fundamental role of the doctor in protecting patients from harm. There is no room for doubt - if one has grounds to believe that a healthcare professional may be putting patients at risk then immediate steps must be taken to flag up the concerns to an appropriate individual. If there is uncertainty, advice should be sought.

Unfortunately the development of a no-blame environment has not yet been achieved so that there remains significant concerns in the minds of those who have to consider flagging up examples of poor practice. So-called whistle blowers will be concerned that anxieties will be inappropriately investigated and may lead to draconian sanctions and public exposure being heaped upon their colleague. Issues raised by past experiences lead to the conclusion that current processes for investigating and dealing with poor performance are often far from perfect.

Problems with dealing with poor performance

- The present medical disciplinary procedures are not entirely coherent and are punishment-based.
- The line of responsibility into management (responsibility for clinical matters ultimately rests with the organisation's Chief Executive) can lead to the procedures being interpreted and applied in a manner which seeks to protect the organisation as the primary goal.
- Practitioners, under the threat of formal suspension, can accept informal processes, such as voluntary ('gardening') leave and thus leave themselves in a limbo which is not covered by the procedures themselves.
- Sound methodology for investigating and assessing possible poor performance is lacking.

Within single NHS organisations, be they primary or secondary care organisations, huge responsibilities rest with the chief executive, medical director, director of nursing and director of human resources. An effective approach to detecting and managing poor performance will only develop if those individuals put appropriate structures in place.

However, policies and structures alone will be inadequate if confidence in these individuals is lacking. One approach to building confidence is to have ready access to independent advice for these key people. This can be provided both from within the organisation and from external agencies such as the NCAA. It is clear that the days of the 'three wise men' are over; independent advice must come from those who have been trained appropriately.

Training requirements for those dealing with poor performance

◆ Knowledge of the legal context of performance issues.

◆ Insight into the evolving methodologies for assessing clinical practice.

◆ An understanding of the options for managing problems with professional interpersonal relationships and dysfunctional behaviour.

◆ Knowledge of the role of Occupational Health services in assessing and helping those with health problems that are impacting on performance.

One of the most common causes of breakdown in clinical systems is the individual who is seen to be dysfunctional or difficult. This may manifest itself in many ways but is characterised by difficulty in working in the context of the wider clinical team. Historically such people's eccentricities and conflicts have been tolerated but there is now recognition that their behaviour does generate risks to patients even if they are performing at a high clinical level. The culture of healthcare is changing so that such dysfunction is more likely nowadays to be identified and challenged.

The difficulty that arises is in finding mechanisms that will address the problems that present themselves and resolve disputes without losing the individuality and clinical strengths of the person in question. Where such dysfunction is posing problems it is important to identify the difficulty early, before it escalates. The medical director, nursing director or human resources director are appropriate individuals to tackle such issues. Input from sources external to the organisation may be needed in order to engage people in a process that might resolve the issues that have arisen.

Much good progress can be made in tackling difficult situations early with under-performing colleagues using some of the approaches above. But many will also know of situations where the problem seems utterly intractable. A colleague who, despite all professional help, remedial support and supportive management effort, remains a problem and a worry. Perhaps clinical governance doesn't offer any other solutions in such situations. It may have its own limits of power and persuasion.

It could be argued therefore that one of the most important skills to be developed by those healthcare professionals with responsibilities for managing poor performance is recognising when the 'softly softly' line has failed and the need for immediate management action has been reached to protect patient safety. Taking the decision to opt for the hard-nosed approach such as disciplinary action and/or referral to the relevant regulatory body will never be easy.

References

1   Reason JT. Chapter 1. *Clinical Risk Management.* Vincent C (Ed). BMJ Books, London.

2   North American Symptomatic Carotid Endarterectomy Trial Collaborators. Benefit of carotid endarterectomy in patients with symptomatic moderate or severe stenosis. *N Engl J Med* 1988; 339: 1415-25.

3   European Carotid Surgery Trialists Collaborative Group. Randomised trial of endarterectomy for recently symptomatic carotid stenosis: final results of the MRC European Carotid Surgery Trial (ESCT). *The Lancet* 1998; 351: 1379-87.

4   Secker-Walker J, Taylor-Adams S. Clinical Incident Reporting. In: *Clinical Risk Management: Enhancing Patient Safety, 2nd Ed.* Vincent C (Ed). BMJ Books, London, 2001: 431.

5   Good Medical Practice. General Medical Council, London, 1998.

Further reading

•   Seeking Patients' Consent: the ethical considerations. Nov 1998. www.gmc-uk.org/standards/CONSENT.htm.

•   BAMM Clinical Directors Series: Clinical Governance Day by Day. British Association of Medical Managers, 2001.

•   When Things Go Wrong. Association of Trust Medical Directors Disciplinary Resource Pack, 1997.

•   Reason J. Human error: models and management. *BMJ* 2000; 320: 768-770.

•   Department of Health. An organisation with a memory: report of an expert group on learning from adverse events in the NHS. The Stationery Office, London, 2000.

•   Department of Health. Building a safer NHS for patients. The Stationery Office, London, 2001.

•   National Patient Safety Agency. Doing Less Harm. NPSA, London, 2001.

•   Department of Health. External Inquiry into the adverse incident that occurred at Queen's Medical Centre, Nottingham, 4th January 2001. The Stationery Office, London, 2001.

•   National Clinical Assessment Authority. Handbook for Hospital and Community Health Services. London, 2002.

Chapter 14

Clinical audit

The nice thing about standards is that there are so many to choose from.
Andres S Tannenbaum

A brief history of audit

The idea of medical audit is not new. The Charter of the Royal College of Physicians of 1518 has a reference to audit and states that one of the College's functions is to uphold the standards of medicine "both for their own honour and public benefit" [1].

When the Medical Act of 1858 [2] established the General Medical Council (GMC) to regulate the medical profession on behalf of the state, there was an implicit expectation that the profession was to self-regulate the quality of clinical care. Self-regulation remained largely in the hands of the profession, through the GMC, when the NHS was created in 1948.

Recognisable medical audit has taken place throughout the health service for many years and some early audits, such as the Confidential Enquiry into Maternal Deaths, which began in 1951, continue today. It has also long been the practice of many clinicians to monitor their own work in relation to complications and deaths on both an individual basis and within the more formal surroundings of hospital mortality and morbidity meetings. Individual enthusiasts undertook much of the early audit work and those who did not wish to participate were under no obligation to do so.

Throughout the 1980s, however, there was increasing interest from both within the medical profession and from politicians in the concept of audit and its potential to generate clinical quality improvement. This reflected general concerns about quality performance within public services in general, which was a prominent theme of the decade.

Medical audit in the NHS

Then, in 1989, the Conservative Government's NHS reforms were revealed. The development of the purchaser/provider split and General Practitioner (GP) fundholding grabbed the headlines but, in addition, the reforms contained a commitment to developing medical audit as a lever for change and improvement. The details of the plans for audit were given in one of a series of working papers: *Working for Patients: Medical Audit - working paper 6*.

This paper set out plans for a comprehensive system of medical audit, covering both primary and secondary care. It was explicit that all healthcare providers in the NHS should develop medical audit programmes involving medical staff in reviewing standards of care and practice. The benefits of the audit programme were expected to be profound and wide ranging. A cash injection of £221 million was made to facilitate the process.

An internal discussion paper in the Department of Health at that time stated:

"Medical audit should trigger changes in practice within specialties, across specialties, across provider units and across boundaries including those between primary, secondary and tertiary care. The findings of medical audit should encourage comparison and challenge working practices throughout the NHS..... This should result in optimal delivery of effective and appropriate care by the right professionals, in the right combination, in the right setting and at the right time. " [3]

Critics of the Conservative reforms would argue that they represented a massive gamble of an experiment. Where was the evidence that introducing a pseudo-competitive market into healthcare would ever deliver significant efficiency gains? Similarly, the heavy reliance on audit as a vehicle for quality improvement was based on conjecture rather than positive experience from other healthcare systems. With hindsight, it is now appreciated that medical audit on its own was never capable of producing its anticipated benefits. Perhaps because this attempt to implement formal medical audit in the NHS was wrapped up in the wider and unpopular NHS reforms, there was genuine professional concern that the methodology was wrong. Where were the time, interest, skills, data and information technology (IT) systems going to come from? Were patients actually going to benefit from the process? Could the money be better used elsewhere in direct patient care?

Evolution of clinical audit

It did not take long for the limitations of audit undertaken solely within the medical profession to become clear. The experience of the generation of clinicians that lived through this particular audit era was one of frustration. The audit process itself too often proved cumbersome and frustrating, while the obligatory audit meetings were of distinctly variable quality. It was therefore clear that the medical audit process had an obvious need for a phase of evolution and refinement. Multi-disciplinary approaches to audit were developed and the term 'clinical audit' was born.

As thinking around audit crystallised and people became more realistic about the capabilities of data measurement, the inability of the process to effect change by itself became clear. Audit was no longer being seen as the central mechanism for improving the quality of healthcare but as one tool in an altogether more complex process of quality assurance.

Impact of the clinical governance agenda

When plans for clinical governance were announced in 1997, clinical audit formed part of a modernisation package for the NHS. Audit was promoted as a valuable tool that would contribute towards the required improvement in the quality of care and, for the first time, professional participation within the process became a requirement rather than an expectation [4].

This sudden weight of responsibility placed on healthcare professionals came with the recognition that external support would be required if audit was to be used to best effect. Support was to come in the form of external organisations with responsibility for developing national standards against which we could effectively compare our practice. In addition, the time commitment required for effective audit (as well as other clinical governance requirements) was recognised. Recognition without delivery of a solution to the problem of actually finding the necessary time, however, means that this promise of support appears to be only partially grounded in reality.

Defining clinical audit

Audit has been defined by Irvine and Irvine as [5]:

"The method used by health professionals to assess, evaluate, and improve the care of patients in a systematic way, to enhance their health and quality of life."

The current concept and practice of clinical audit was explored in a paper commissioned by the recent Public Inquiry into Children's Heart Surgery at the Bristol Royal Infirmary. It stated:

To health professionals, audit offers a systematic framework for investigating and assessing their work and for introducing and monitoring improvements. The process of carrying out an audit involves a characteristic sequence of events which includes:

◆ Defining standards, criteria, targets or protocols for good practice against which performance can be compared.

◆ Gathering systematic and objective evidence about performance.

◆ Comparing results against standards and/or among peers.

◆ Identifying deficiencies and taking action to remedy them.

◆ Monitoring the effects of this action i.e. "closing the audit loop". [6]

This cycle of events is frequently represented pictorially (Figure 1).

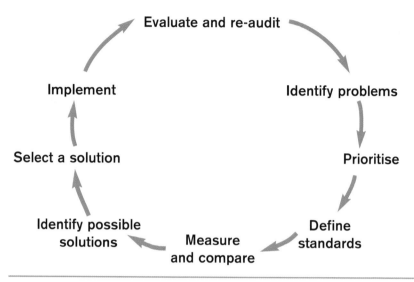

Figure 1. The audit cycle.

Terminology

Even today, despite the wealth of literature and recent high profile cases, the term 'audit' is still often misused within the health service. It is still common for junior doctors to present audits of individual consultant's practice or local departmental findings in relation to a new or interesting technique. Such audits often use small patient numbers, without pre-prescribed standards for comparison and have no intention for effecting change.

Practical suggestions

- Understand what clinical audit is and is not.
- Show your outline audit project to your Trust's clinical audit team and get advice before you start.
- Share a good (i.e. well-conducted) audit with colleagues in other hospitals.

Lack of audit training

It is now a requirement for all healthcare professionals to be involved in regular clinical audit. Training assessment portfolios for junior doctors and, more recently, consultants include a section for audit. The Joint Committee on Higher Surgical and Medical Training state that [7]:

"Ongoing commitment to audit is essential and clear documentation of those projects should be present in the portfolio".

Additionally, medical job application forms now also include a section related to audit; this section carries a significant number of short-listing points for applications.

Despite the requirements for health professionals to be, and to be seen to be, actively involved in the process, very little training and on-going education in clinical audit currently exists. Some Trusts regularly include audit training for their junior doctors at the beginning of the twice yearly changeover, but attendance is generally unregulated and there are no sanctions against those who do not participate.

For those doctors who qualified before the 1990s, education and training in audit existed only sporadically. Historically, doctors were

---

Practical suggestions

- Don't presume you are skilled in audit - make sure you are!
- Attend a formal audit training course run by your local Trust or Deanery.
- If no training course exists, invite someone from your audit department to do a teaching session within a departmental meeting.
- Plan and undertake an audit, taking advice from your Trust's audit team and use the skills you have learnt.
- Don't revert to old habits, which we know, die hard.
- Be prepared to challenge 'audits' that are not really audits at all.

responsible for carrying out their own audits and it was generally assumed that the medical profession would have the inherent skills to carry out effective clinical audit. This was not always the case. There are countless examples of inadequate audit undertaken by medical professionals across the country.

Identifying audit topics

Finding a suitable topic for audit is the first potential pitfall in the process of conducting a useful audit. Audits can be grouped into three distinct categories: audit of outcome, audit of process and audit of structure. These may be combined in single audit projects when a broad evaluation of care is being conducted.

Audit categories

We can use diabetes care as an example:

- **Audit of outcome** eg. rates of microvascular and macrovascular complications or HbA1c levels in patients.
- **Audit of process** eg. comprehensiveness of annual recall procedures and examination.
- **Audit of structure** eg. numbers of nurse specialists, presence of a diabetes register.

Ideally no audit should be done that does not look at some aspect of patient outcome. But in many circumstances this is not always possible. If there is solid evidence that certain aspects of the process of healthcare result in good outcomes then it is reasonable to concentrate on the process of care as a compromise instead. An audit that looks purely at the structure of care and ignores process and outcome measures is likely to be of passing interest only in terms of promoting improvements in care.

Up to the present time, audits have typically been undertaken because of the particular interests and enthusiasms of the clinical team. While there is nothing inherently wrong with this approach, it is immediately limiting in terms of fulfilling the requirements of clinical governance. The philosophy behind clinical governance calls for a different, and less comfortable, starting point: the question is not so much "What is the team good at?" but "Where might our deficiencies lie?". One way of meeting this challenge is to consider one's attitude to the audit. If the results are eagerly awaited in view of an expectation of self-congratulation, then perhaps the topic was poorly selected; on the other hand, a slight feeling of anxiety ahead of the outcome being revealed probably points to a worthwhile audit having been undertaken.

Practical suggestions

- Use known clinical risk areas (eg. in your Trust's risk register) as good topics for audit eg. infection control, drug errors.
- Identify patterns arising out of complaints/critical incident reporting to focus audit work.
- Don't re-invent the wheel - use existing audits that have been road tested in other hospitals in similar specialities and so cut out the hard work in designing the project/data collection. You will also be able to compare easily how you are doing compared to others outside your hospital. Nationally run audits eg. through the Royal Colleges are a good way of getting involved with a relative minimum of fuss.
- Don't try to perform an audit on conditions with low patient numbers in your Trust. You will need to collaborate with other Trusts if this is to be worthwhile.

Defining/setting standards

No audit should be initiated without a clear definition of the ideal 'good practice' criteria which will form the baseline comparator and an understanding as to what would hope to be achieved in terms of local standards. By agreeing the criteria at the outset, there will be clarity as to what data need to be collected and, importantly, what information is not required.

Practical suggestions

- The criteria of ideal practice should be defined, where at all possible, by a national body or a recognised peer expert group. You, however, may want to agree what your own local standards are within these criteria given the practicalities of delivering the care in your own particular Trust setting.
- Make sure that the literature has been carefully searched for evidence of best practice before getting underway.
- Get trained in how to use the internet for literature searching through your Trust librarian.
- Become familiar with the National Electronic Library for Health (www.nelh.nhs.uk) as a World Wide Web gateway to the best knowledge systems in healthcare today. It includes access to the Cochrane register and database, OVID databases, NICE guidance and guidelines, the National Clinical Governance Support Unit, the BMJ's Clinical Evidence resource and much more.
- On the same site is published guidance on best practice in clinical audit for those wanting to learn more on audit methodology (www.nelh.nhs.uk/nice_bpca.asp).

Data collection and databases

It is immediately apparent that effective audit relies on accurate and relevant data being accessible. As previously noted, all too often in the NHS there is a basic failing in the systems that collect and record information. The result of this defect is that reliable information is frequently only obtained if time-consuming manual trawls of lists, registers or patients' notes are undertaken. It is therefore important to decide at an early stage whether the time and effort that is going to be expended on data collection will bring sufficient reward by answering an important question with a degree of reliability; a preliminary statistical power calculation may help in this decision-making process.

In view of the difficulties with data acquisition, it is appropriate to plan ahead and decide what information collection should be built into patterns of clinical care. Should the diabetic clinic be run in a way that allows results and complications to be logged onto a database in real time?

The national NHS strategy, *Information for Health* [8], recognises these difficulties and aims to tackle the issue. But inevitably it will take many years before clinicians feel that information technology and patient administration systems are designed to encompass a reliable and useful functionality that supports clinical audit.

Practical suggestions

- Use standard database software eg. Microsoft Excel/Access so that others can use the database easily in the future for re-audit.
- When designing your data collection, set up your IT database at the same time and use 'dummy' data to work out what analysis you really need for the audit. In doing so you can eliminate unnecessary data collection fields and make sure you are clear at the outset what the audit is really measuring.
- If you are sampling patient notes, check out with your Trust's clinical audit team whether your sample size is big enough to measure meaningful changes between this and future repeat audits.
- Have a system where completed audit database files are kept for future reference in repeat audits.
- Be aware of your responsibilities regarding data protection.

Creating improvement through audit

The high aspirations that accompanied the development of clinical audit in the NHS were built on the assumption that participation in audit would automatically lead to improvements in healthcare delivery. Unfortunately quality gains have been found to be far more elusive than might have been imagined. Audit itself should have been audited to see whether the resources being invested were being used to the maximum advantage. How can the best be brought out of audit?

Firstly, a significant problem exists in relation to the thorny issue of unfinished audit projects and the lack of repeat audits. The audit department within our Trust recently calculated that 40% of audits that were initiated were never completed. There are multiple reasons for this, but prominent is the involvement of junior doctors who might not have adequate time or the inclination to finish the project within the time frame of their job within the Trust. The pressure for junior doctors to be involved in audit comes both from the requirement to build up the individual curriculum vitae (with a view to passing exams and gaining future employment) and at a departmental level where there is desire on the part of individual consultants to have their work reviewed systematically without the time or resource to undertake this themselves.

A second issue relates to audit choice and design. It is appropriate to consider, at the time when the project is being set up, what changes might be made if a particular outcome emerges. If results point to a substandard service should patients be referred to a different team or does the result enable a strong case for more resources to be deployed? Inevitably, if an audit is chosen that is instinctively uncomfortable for staff (i.e. there is a likelihood that current practice is below standard), then there maybe more chance of seeing change result.

An additional aspect of design that impacts on the likely benefit of an audit is the involvement of individuals from different disciplines. Would an audit of the quality of clinical notes be more effective if it was carried out with the involvement of secretarial and other administrative staff? If the performance of a clinical team is being assessed then the whole team should have the ability to influence and participate in the audit process.

However, it would be wrong not to acknowledge the extent to which audit can be a vehicle for benefit. Many audit projects in their own right result in useful change simply because someone has taken the trouble to define good practice and shares this knowledge across the clinical team: audit should be intrinsically educational. Additionally, the process of collecting data can be beneficial as it points out any deficiencies in the routine recording and handling of clinical information. These beneficial spin-offs from the actual audit process itself arise even as the audit is being undertaken.

The fundamental rationale behind clinical audit is that improvements will arise as a result of completion of the audit cycle. In simple terms, the audit demonstrates the need for change, the change is made and benefits are seen ..... sorted! Unfortunately, changes in working practices and clinical behaviour are not easily made. It is all too common for a problem to be identified only for the same issue to emerge again after an interval - perhaps because a change of team personnel has taken place. Careful thought and the use of project management techniques may be needed before the topic can be finally said to have been dealt with effectively.

Practical suggestions

- Create a 3 or 5 yearly audit plan for your department with an annual review on progress.
- Use a project initiation form prior to the commencement of each new audit to improve its impact (Appendix III).
- Identify a non-clinical member of the department to manage the programme and chase up progress.
- Summarise annual progress in a brief report to the Trusts's Clinical Governance Sub-Committee and/or Clinical Audit Team.
- Delegate senior members of the clinical team to have responsibility for individual audit areas and allocate junior staff to support each project as they rotate through the department.
- Have at least three departmental sessions each year where the most recently completed audits are discussed and action points agreed.

References

1   The Charter of Incorporation. Granted by Henry VIII to the President and College, or Commonalty, of the Faculty of Physic in London. Sept 23rd 1518. In: *The Charter and Bye-Laws.* Including Regulations and Resolutions. The Royal College of Physicians of London, Jan 1995.

2   The New Medical Act with explanatory notes for the guidance of the medical practitioner & student. Robert Mortimer Glover, James Bridge Davidson, London 1858.

3   Medical and Clinical Audit. Chapter 18. Annex A. The Bristol Royal Infirmary Inquiry.

4   The New NHS, Modern, Dependable. Secretary of State for Health. The Stationery Office, London, December 1997.

5   Irvine D, Irvine S. *Making Sense of Audit.* Radcliffe Medical Press, Oxford, 1991.

6   Hughes J, Humphrey C. Medical audit in general practice. King's Fund, London, 1990.

7   JCHST website. Contents of training portfolio. March 2001. Communications Document. Available at www.jchst.org.

8   Information For Health - 1. An Information Strategy for the modern NHS. NHS Information Authority. Available at www.nhsia.nhs.uk.

Further reading

•   National Institute for Clinical Excellence. *Principles for Best Practice in Clinical Audit.* Radcliffe Medical Press, Oxford, 2002.

•   Morrell C, Harvey G. *The Clinical Audit Handbook.* Balliere Tindall, London, 1999.

Chapter 15

Research & development

Medicinal discovery
It moves in mighty leaps
It leapt straight past the common cold
And gave it us for keeps.
Pam Ayres

Practising evidence-based medicine

The application of the philosophy, which has driven the development of clinical governance, strongly supports the drive towards a scientific approach to medical practice. The direction of travel is towards evidence-based medicine, which creates an environment where unsubstantiated professional opinion is questioned and tested. It can, of course, be argued that medicine has always had strong scientific roots; what is new are the supporting structures that are trying to ensure that scientific knowledge is both available and acted upon.

Requirements for evidence-based practice

◆ Knowledge of the options that might be available in a given situation.
◆ Having relevant information readily to hand - preferably at the point of consultation.
◆ Interpreting the data in the clinical context.
◆ Discussing the possible choice of interventions with the patient.

The drive towards an evidence-based approach should provide the NHS with a degree of reliability and uniformity, both highly desired commodities within a comprehensive service. It is well recognised that most healthcare systems will generate significant variations in the quality of different services. The expectation is that a more structured and prescriptive approach, across the NHS, will do much to reduce this variation. The potential disadvantage of clipping the wings of innovative clinical teams is perhaps a price worth paying. Those that wish to push at the frontiers can still do so, but they have to make progress through research and development processes which themselves have high standards of governance.

Unfortunately, although laudable, the development of an evidence-based approach is not without its difficulties. Perhaps the most obvious difficulty arises from the fact that reliable evidence is so difficult to obtain; even where randomised controlled trial data are available, a completely convincing conclusion may have to await a meta-analysis of several such studies. But, for most areas of medicine, far lower quality information is all that is available. A second issue relates to the fact that published data usually relate to subsets of the clinical population. The conclusions that a study might draw may be correct for the group studied, but extrapolation of the results to other populations, may be inappropriate. It is often the very young, the elderly and those with multiple pathologies who are not covered by the evidence-base. Other effects must point towards a cautious approach to evidence. The phenomenon, which results in patients who participate in clinical trials having better outcomes than those whose care is conducted outside such studies, is well recognised.

However, the individual clinician is faced with further problems in this area. Too little evidence is often accompanied by too much information. Those who are trying to gather the evidence-base to provide patients with high quality care are constantly bombarded with reports on new techniques and interventions, from professional journals, royal colleges, government publications, websites, pharmaceutical and equipment companies and the media. In such an environment it can be very difficult to know where to look for the best and most reliable information.

The foundation of evidence

An understanding of research processes is vital for those who are trying to make headway with evidence-based practice. Research is the foundation of the evidence that we seek. Without insight into research methodology, there is little chance of an individual being able to appropriately interpret the data they may have assembled. Their patient may suffer as a result.

While we maintain responsibility for treating patients in our roles as healthcare professionals, we must recognise and act on our responsibility for gaining and appropriately applying the evidence on which we base our practice. With this in mind, it follows that we should all understand when evidence should be incorporated into our practice, when its results should be observed over time and when it should be digested and rejected as poor evidence. No individual working in the NHS today has the time, resources or energy to investigate for themselves every aspect of their practice. However, each of us can learn and apply techniques to help us make increasingly intelligent use of the research evidence available.

Clinical governance advises us that we should continuously improve the quality of our service by understanding how we best use the research of others and how to undertake research ourselves ethically (also known as research governance). By doing this we can be confident we are moving in the required direction.

Gathering and assessing clinical evidence

All healthcare professionals will search for established evidence far more often than they ever undertake research for themselves. Yet little emphasis is placed upon this activity and its ability to impact on clinical quality.

There are two aspects to data gathering: knowing where to look and knowing how to assess the evidence that is unearthed.

Practising evidence-based medicine

The methodology that allows an evidence-based approach to be adopted is becoming increasingly sophisticated. The essential steps are as follows:

♦ **Formulate the question** Relevant information will only be obtained if the correct information is put into the search engines being used. Patient characteristics (age, sex, co-morbidity etc.) and the intervention under consideration (diagnostic, therapeutic) must be correctly presented if useful evidence is to emerge.

♦ **Find the evidence** The key elements are to select the database resources and to establish appropriate search strategies.

♦ **Analyse the evidence** Sifting the evidence and assessing its relevance and strength is aided by the application of grading systems. Evidence hierarchies establish levels of confidence in the conclusions that have been drawn based on the source of the evidence (eg. systematic reviews, meta-analyses, randomised controlled trials, case series and, lastly, expert opinion). Similarly, there is a grading system for the recommendations that emerge from such information.

♦ **Apply the evidence** It is critical to the evidence-based process that the conclusions emerging from the process are not applied unthinkingly to the clinical situation in question. The aim is to marry clinical expertise with the best available, relevant information which can help to guide decision-making.

♦ **Evaluate and audit the process** Where major changes in practice have been made it may be appropriate to audit the effectiveness of the development.

There are numerous Internet resources relating to this topic. The Centre for Evidence-Based Medicine can be found at: www.cebm.net.

Knowing where to look will always be dependent on what type of evidence you are looking for, but there are some key on-line databases which are of exceptional value (see Appendix I). The National Electronic Library for Health is a good place to start the search process (www.nelh.nhs.uk).

Assessing the evidence available is a complex and sophisticated process. Some personal experience of research is invaluable in generating insight into this field. Recognition of the pitfalls relating to evidence interpretation leads to the conclusion that original data are of most use to those who have a particular interest and expertise in an area of practice. When looking at topics that fall outside such areas, it is sensible to look for reviews that have been conducted by recognised authorities; the indigestible raw evidence is then at least partly processed for consumption.

Practical suggestions

- Make use of the skills and experience of your Trust librarians - they are familiar with the new electronic knowledge systems.
- Contact your local public health department for help and support - consultants/specialists in public health are trained in these skills.
- Go on a critical appraisal/evidence-based medicine course.
- Maintain an active journal club within the department.
- Find a useful (and easily remembered) tool to critique research papers.

Responsibilities in undertaking personal research

Research is traditionally viewed as a worthy activity that generates advantage to patients and esteem to the researcher. However, this

Key responsibilities in research governance

Principal investigator and other researchers
- Developing proposals that are ethical and seeking ethics committee approval.
- Conducting research to the agreed protocol and in accordance with legal requirements and guidance.
- Ensuring participant welfare while in the study.
- Feeding back results of research to participants.

Local research ethics committee
- Ensuring that the proposed research is ethical and respects the dignity, rights, safety and well-being of participants.

Sponsor
- Assuring the scientific quality of proposed research.
- Ensuring research ethics committee approval has been sought.
- Ensuring arrangements are in place for the management and monitoring of research.

Employing organisation
- Promoting a quality research culture.
- Ensuring researchers understand and discharge their responsibilities.
- Taking responsibility for ensuring the research is properly managed and monitored.

Care organisation/responsible care professional
- Ensuring that research using their patients, users, carers or staff meets the standards set out in the research governance framework.
- Ensuring research ethics committee approval is obtained for all research.
- Retaining responsibility for the care of research participants.

perception is being replaced by a more critical appraisal of research efforts. This shift has come about as research activity comes under greater scrutiny. Lifting this particular stone has unearthed such issues as variable ethical standards, concerns over research's financial environment and problems with fraudulent research. When healthcare research goes wrong, enormous distress and even harm can result for those involved in the project. In order to protect firstly, the research subjects and secondly, ourselves as researchers, it is vital that any research is conducted to high scientific and ethical standards.

These standards are now clearly set out in the government document *Research Governance Framework for Health and Social Care*. All those involved in research should understand their responsibilities within this framework and discharge them appropriately.

Practical suggestions

- Get involved in a sponsored multi-centre trial. This is an excellent way of learning about good research governance as there is a wealth of experience in such trials to guide you through the process of good research practice.
- Consider inviting a member of the Local Research Ethics Committee to a departmental meeting.
- Make contact with the Trust's Research and Development Committee who will have information about research governance.

Research motivation

Published work is inter-linked with professional prestige. This relationship is quite justified when discoveries that will significantly impact on healthcare are disseminated in written form. Unfortunately, the drive for publication as evidence of prestige and career progression can lead to research being carried out with the wrong underlying motivation. Amidst this scramble for papers, and perhaps letters after their names, healthcare professionals can be at risk of falling into the trap of producing "so what?" research. This is research for publication's sake. Depending on the status of the professional meeting or journal involved, the research may not even get aired and is, in any case, unlikely to be of lasting value. We are required to produce quality work in all aspects of our everyday clinical care; research endeavours should reach similar standards.

Study design

It is essential, before embarking on any planned research, to ask the fundamental question "does this matter?". If the topic being examined is inappropriate, no matter how high the quality of the study design, methodology or presentation, people are still going to ask why the research was ever started. This is not a position in which to be found. However, the assessment of what is worthwhile in terms of a research question is not always a straightforward process. Those at the beginning of their professional careers will find this evaluation particularly difficult due to an absence of experienced clinical impression and a lack of in-depth subject knowledge. The fact that the most cited 15% of articles account for 50% of all citations does little to counter the contention that much published research is of minimal value [1].

A thorough literature search is the undoubted starting place for any quality research. It is usual to find that subjects have been broached to a greater or lesser degree within the published literature. But it is rare for there not to be significant unanswered questions within a given medical field. However, there must be genuine doubt as to the answer of a particular question if the project is to be fundamentally ethical; patients cannot be invited to participate in a study that puts subjects into a group which will receive care that is known to be sub-optimal.

High quality, ethical research can only be carried out if care is taken with the design of the study. Sloppy thinking at this stage will have a major negative impact on the outcome of the research effort. A written protocol is essential and it must clearly state the hypothesis to be tested. Having established with clarity what is being examined, it is then necessary for the study to be both designed and powered to be able to accept or reject the hypothesis. There is an ethical requirement on the researcher only to enter subjects into a study that has a realistic prospect of reaching a valid conclusion.

Of course, study design issues reach beyond the requirement to address the primary hypothesis, as a well-founded project will gain added value from its ability to address issues in appropriate detail. For example, quality of life data might not be felt to be essential for a study but could help to throw additional light on patients' response to an intervention.

Practical suggestions

- All hospital libraries will provide help with thorough literature searching.
- Don't stick to your original research question if it has already been answered.
- Make sure that there is a genuine gap in our knowledge - and one that can usefully be addressed.
- Preliminary trials abound - do you have time and resources to undertake a definitive trial?
- Ask colleagues - if in doubt about a research proposal, run it by a number of colleagues who are experienced in research and have time to think about the proposal with you.

Research protocol format

◆ **Title** This should be brief and informative.

◆ **Summary or abstract** About 250 words stating the purpose of the research, describing the study design and methods, and outlining the expected findings. Also included in this section should be the names, qualifications and contact details of the researchers.

◆ **Background and rationale of the study** Describe succinctly the health issue to be addressed. The main research question should be stated clearly, as well as where the research proposal fits in to the current literature surrounding the topic.

◆ **Aims and objectives** Clear primary (and secondary, if appropriate) objectives are needed.

◆ **Experimental design and methods** This should be written in such a way that another person could repeat your study in exactly the same way. This section therefore needs to include:

➤ *Number of subjects/cases - a power calculation is imperative.*

➤ *How the subjects will be selected and over what time period.*

➤ *Subject inclusion/exclusion criteria.*

➤ *How the subjects will be recruited and consented and what information they will be given to help them decide whether to participate.*

➤ *Study type.*

➤ *Procedures/interventions to be carried out (tests, investigations, drugs).*

➤ *Exactly what data will be collected.*

➤ *The methods of data collection should be described (patient questionnaire/instrument) - include information on the reliability and validity of the method.*

➤ *Data analysis techniques to be used.*

◆ **Funding** Detail how the project is going to be financially supported. This is important when submitting a proposal for approval to either the Trust Research and Development Committee or the Local Research Ethics Committee as there is little point approving research that will evidently never be completed due to absence of funding.

◆ **Publication/Presentation aims** What audience is the work aimed to benefit and how will it be presented to them?

Ethical approval

The primary responsibility for the ethical conduct of research lies, of course, with the researchers themselves and their employing Trust. However, the supporting regulatory mechanisms are based on the network of ethics committees. Every NHS organisation works under the umbrella of a Local Research Ethics Committee (LREC), which includes both expert and lay members. The committees are recognised by the Department of Health in their role as independent reviewers of research ethics undertaken within the NHS. The primary responsibility of LRECs is to act in the interests of potential research subjects and communities in protecting dignity, rights, safety and well-being, as described in the document *Research Governance Framework for Health and Social Care*. They should also take into account the interests, needs and safety of researchers who are trying to undertake research of good quality. However, the goals of the researchers will always be a lesser priority for LRECs than the well-being of the study participants.

If a research study will involve work that spans five or more LREC areas then an application for ethical approval should be made to the regional Multi-centre Research Ethics Committee (MREC). There is still a

Research requiring LREC approval

Formal LREC approval for a research project is needed if the research involves [2]:

◆ NHS patients and users (recruited by virtue of their past or present use of the NHS). This includes NHS patients treated under contracts with the private sector.

◆ Foetal material and *in vitro* fertilisation involving NHS patients.

◆ Those who recently died on NHS premises.

◆ Access to records of past and present NHS patients.

◆ The use of, or potential access to, NHS premises or facilities (including NHS staff).

requirement to apply to each of the involved LRECs but the submission is simplified and the procedures more streamlined.

One area of significant practical difficulty is that of separating research from audit. This is particularly important when looked at from the governance point of view; different support and regulatory mechanisms exist for the two activities and failure to apply appropriate standards to one's efforts is a potentially serious professional matter. If in doubt, consult experienced colleagues and have a low threshold for taking soundings from the chairpersons of the Trust's Research and Development Committee (see below) or of the LREC.

The responsibility of the researcher and the LREC do not end when an application is approved. There is a requirement to provide progress reports on the research project and a final communication on completion of the work. Whilst carrying out the research project, any worrying adverse event that occurs, which could be related to the intervention that is part of the study, will also need to be reported to the LREC in case a decision is needed to halt the research study.

It is also important to appreciate that research approval is needed from the host Trust. In general, Trusts will take particular interest in issues of facilities, resource and finance. Arrangements for approval will vary from organisation to organisation but are most commonly directed through a Research and Development Committee prior to a formal submission to the LREC.

Confronting public perceptions of research

Following recent health scandals in Bristol and Alder Hey, Liverpool, the public has become increasingly suspicious of the health system. This does not mean that the public does not appreciate the need for research to be undertaken, or that they are no longer willing participants in the research process. Indeed the public inquiries into both Bristol [3] and Alder Hey [4] found the public accepts the need for medical research and gives it full backing. What is not acceptable to the public is the cloak of professional secrecy and that has surrounded much research into new interventions in the past. Openness and consent is the key to the future for public confidence in health research.

Practical suggestions

- Be aware that the patient/relative/carer you are speaking to may have certain fearful perceptions about research, based on what they have previously heard or experienced. Patients need to have the realities of the proposed research explained to them very carefully, in language that they can understand.
- Be willing to explain any research proposal to patients at length.
- See patients with a relative or friend - four ears are always better than two.
- Always have an information sheet for patients to take away with them, which covers exactly what you are proposing to do.
- Don't expect every patient to consent to your research and give them ample opportunity to say no - it is much easier to continue recruitment than to deal with a study full of non-compliant patients.
- Look at other patient information sheets, particularly those from multi-centre trials. They are always set out in excellent detail and will provide all the points that you need to include in your own information sheets.

Analysing data

There are no simple guidelines for easy data analysis, as the shelves of various medical statistical books will testify. And a book such as this on clinical governance, giving guidance on how to produce work of quality, is no place for oversimplification of what is a very complex area. However, poor data handling and analysis remain a major failing in a significant proportion of research and audit projects. Improving the quality of our efforts in this area will therefore depend, in part, on a better appreciation of statistical methodology.

Practical suggestions

- Stick to the original study aims first and foremost - you have to answer the original research question.
- Always ask for help with statistics at the outset from someone qualified - even if it is just to confirm that you are doing the right thing. Making your first contact at the analysis stage will usually result in a firm rebuff!
- Use standard packages - SPSS, Excel. But there are also excellent public domain freeware packages available that cover the majority of database and statistical analytical functions for healthcare research (www.cdc.gov/epiinfo).
- Don't use a statistical technique unless you are sure that it is appropriate to the analysis you are performing.
- Design your database/spreadsheet for all expected data at the outset.
- Do an analysis run using dummy data to test your data collection proforma and clarify your analysis outputs.
- Enter data onto the spreadsheet as you go along - this will prevent any repetitive strain injuries at a later date!

Presenting research

A final, often neglected, responsibility for anyone undertaking research is to produce an end product that effectively disseminates any messages that the work has delivered. What patient would ever give consent to enter a study if they knew the results would never be made available to a wider audience? It is also essential for the work to be presented effectively.

Some work will obviously be more appropriate for departmental or local presentation while other work may benefit a wider audience at a large scientific meeting or through publication. The processes of presenting to different audiences using the varied mediums of writing, podium or poster presentations each have their own challenges and pitfalls.

There is no doubt that some people find presenting easier than others. But there is certainly no great secret to it; presenting is just another skill that must be acquired. Some thought and consideration for your audience will avoid the need to apologise in the middle of a presentation for the slide that is "a bit busy"! The fundamental point of presentation should always be kept at the forefront of your mind - spreading the message of your research findings in a way that the audience can understand and potentially use.

Practical suggestions

- Follow the speaker guidelines and don't presume your presentation is so interesting that you will get away with straying from your instructions.
- Always follow a format
  - ➤ *Introduction (tell them what you're going to tell them).*
  - ➤ *Aims, methods and results (tell them).*
  - ➤ *Conclusions/summary (tell them what you've told them).*
- Keep slides simple - maximum 50 words, maximum 6 lines.
- Don't overdo the PowerPoint - having slides flying in from all angles just distracts from your message.
- Don't just read your slides - they should be a representation of something that you are saying, not the whole talk.
- Use simple graphs and pictures, not just words.
- Practice in front of colleagues and friends!
- Get them to ask you practice questions and incorporate these into your talk if appropriate.

Publishing research

If a piece of research is of sufficient quality it should be published. Thought has to be given, before submission for publication, to the audience it should be aimed at. Choosing the right journal and writing it up in the style of that journal may mean the difference between acceptance and rejection. For a well-planned and designed piece of research the following reasons for rejection should not apply [5]:

Common reasons why papers are rejected for publication

◆ The study did not examine an important scientific issue.

◆ The study was not original.

◆ The study did not actually test the authors' hypothesis.

◆ A different study design should have been used.

◆ Practical difficulties (eg. recruiting subjects) led the authors to compromise on the original protocol.

◆ The sample size was too small.

◆ The study was uncontrolled or inadequately controlled.

◆ The statistical analysis was incorrect or inappropriate.

◆ The authors have drawn unjustified conclusions.

◆ There is considerable conflict of interest (eg. author might benefit financially from publications and insufficient safeguards were seen to be in place to guard against bias).

◆ The paper is so badly written that it is incomprehensible.

◆ The paper was not interesting.

References

1   Seglen PO. Why the impact factor of journals should not be used for evaluating research. *BMJ* 1997; 314: 497.

2   www.corec.org.uk/whentoapply.htm.

3   The Bristol Royal Infirmary Inquiry. July 2001. Available at www.bristol-inquiry.org.uk/final_report.

4   The Royal Liverpool Children's Inquiry. January 2001. Available at www.rlcinquiry.org.uk.

5   Greenhalgh T. *How to read a paper: the basics of evidence-based medicine,* 2nd Ed. BMJ Books, London, 2001.

Further reading

- Research and Development in the NHS - An Introductory Guide. Available at www.hop.man.ac.uk/Academic/researchdevelopment.
- MRC Guidelines for Good Clinical Practice in Clinical Trials available through the R&D pages on the Department of Health website at www.doh.gov.uk/research.
- Statistical guidelines for contributors to medical journals. Chapter 14. In: *Statistics with Confidence.* Altman, Machin, Bryant. BMJ Books, London, 2000.
- Governance Arrangements for NHS Research Ethics Committees. July 2001. Available at www.doh.gov.uk/research/documents/gafrec.doc.
- Oxman AD, Sackett DL, Guyatt GH. Users' guides to the medical literature. I. How to get started. The Evidence-Based Medicine Working Group. *JAMA* 1993; 270: 2093-5 (and subsequent articles in the series).
- Research Governance Framework for Health and Social Care. March 2001. Available at www.doh.gov.uk/research/rd3/nhsrandd/researchgovernance/govhome.htm.

Chapter 16

Staffing and staff management

In order that people may be happy in their work, these three things are needed: they must be fit for it; they must not do too much of it; and they must have a sense of success in it.
John Ruskin

Successful working practices within any part of the NHS are dependent on effective teamwork. A functional team is a prerequisite upon which any drive for continuous improvement rests. Experience in risk management points towards the critical role of team dynamics in determining the outcome of care. It goes without saying that some teams will be easier to work in than others, since colleagues (somewhat like family) may be inflicted upon us rather than chosen! Unfortunately the NHS is no stranger to dysfunctional team-working. We will all have witnessed the destructive effect of such a breakdown in working relationships, and its detrimental effect on both patient care and staff. It is therefore essential that every opportunity be taken to promote and develop co-operative ways of working that will lead to the creation of successful units.

Recruiting staff

Within the current NHS climate, staffing recruitment and retention is a huge issue and the problems are varied. In some areas vacant posts cannot be filled simply because there are no candidates. The most striking example of this today is in nursing. Units are having to advertise worldwide in order to attract candidates; attempts are also being made to attract trained nurses who have left the profession back in to the job. The same is true for many of the new consultant posts that have been created. In contrast there are other areas where the competition for jobs is fierce;

some vacant posts for junior staff lead to a short-listing process involving dozens of applications.

The common goal in these two contrasting situations is the desire to attract the right candidate into the vacancy on offer. Those desperate for a candidate will not wish to lower the required standards and employ someone who is not up to the job. While those with a flood of applicants may find it very difficult to choose the person who is most suitable for the post on offer, as opposed to the candidate who appears most professionally qualified on paper.

It is worth remembering that jobs, and indeed hospitals, have long established reputations; those with a strong reputation will have fewer problems in attracting good candidates. On the other hand, a bad reputation can be difficult to shake off. If nothing is changed, a unit can find itself in a vicious circle where recruitment efforts result in a list of weak candidates who, if appointed, will do nothing to enhance the standing of the department.

Practical suggestions

- Enhance the standard job advert by emphasising something about the department - the opportunity for employees to undertake research projects or support to attend a particular training course.
- Ensure that jobs are advertised at appropriate times for the type of candidate you're after. If an advert is out too late for junior doctors, most good candidates will have found employment elsewhere.
- Take an interest in the short-listing process; you will have no grounds for complaint about the candidates being interviewed if you did not contribute earlier in the process.
- Do your bit for marketing your department in your professional networking - it's all too easy to emphasise the problems and talk down the positive aspects of your situation.
- Court PRHOs who appear to have good potential.
- Support initiatives to make the junior doctors' working and living environment better in your Trust.

The interview process

Interviews are a minefield for both the interviewer and the interviewee. Considerable attention has been paid to the issues surrounding appointments in recent years. Gone are the days when a shared avid interest in rock climbing or rugby was allowed to clinch an appointment. The process has to be fair and be seen to be fair. Fortunately, adherence with employment law will usually be ensured by the involvement of Human Resources personnel in the selection and interview procedure. Furthermore, basic training in relation to the issues surrounding employment is widely available in the form of selection and interviewing courses.

It is self-evident that selection bias in relation to age, gender or ethnic background is unacceptable. However, selection procedures now look to a demonstrable level of fairness beyond these core issues. Documentation in relation to the criteria for judging candidates, reasons for rejection or short listing and the interview itself are essential. Challenges by unsuccessful candidates are no longer exceptional events.

Interviewing is a skill which should not be underestimated. The aim of the interview is to appoint the strongest candidate for the post and should not be abused as an opportunity to wield power inappropriately. The best applicant may turn out not to be the most eloquent and confident individual on parade; some preparation before the interview and sensible lines of questioning are needed in order to expose the underlying qualities of the interviewees.

Finally, it is good practice to provide feedback to unsuccessful candidates. This is not just a question of good manners (although that is clearly a consideration) - it will enable the applicant to improve their chances of a future, successful appointment by addressing any deficiencies that have been exposed by the appointment process.

Practical suggestions

- If you are seeing candidates pre-interview, make an appointment and have their curriculum vitae (CV) available to you. This will appear efficient to those seeking employment and will help you to remember individual candidates.
- If you are keen to sell the position to prospective candidates, arrange for them to look around the department with a current team member who can fill them in on the realities of the job.
- Ensure that you have suitable rooms for the interview and for candidates to wait, with tea and coffee available.
- Ensure that Human Resources staff are available perhaps even to chair the interview panel. This means that you can use their specialist recruitment and selection skills to ensure the interview is conducted successfully and within legal guidelines.
- Keep a record of all questions asked and some notes regarding candidate performance - there is now much greater emphasis placed at all levels on feedback for both successful and unsuccessful candidates.
- Remember that, under equal opportunities law, all candidates must be asked the same questions.
- Gather opinion from all others involved in the interview and don't presume that you have picked up on everything that has been said (or not said) during the course of the interviews. Too often a member of staff from human resources is present at interview for administrative purposes without their experience and views being fully utilised.
- Go on a recruitment and selection training course. It will make you a much better interviewer and give potential candidates more confidence that you know what you are doing.

Retaining staff

Maintaining a pleasant and productive work environment is key to staff retention. As healthcare professionals we have no power over salary and are therefore unable to offer financial incentives to individuals threatening to leave their posts. It is important to look at other reasons why individuals should choose to leave if we are to have any influence over their choice to do so. Addressing any problems before a decision to leave is reached may avoid the upheaval that surrounds losing a key member of the team. Staff may leave jobs that they enjoy due to life changes, which no longer fit into their current working arrangements. Childcare issues are a common source of difficulty and consideration of requests for flexible training or job-sharing may allow the individual to remain in the unit.

There are individuals who also wish to work reduced hours in order to pursue other interests or employment opportunities, or simply for the quality of life that it brings. Such requests should never be dismissed out of hand, but considered carefully in the cold light of day. Once again, there is a need to take advice from the Human Resources department, as they will be familiar with the practicalities of flexible working patterns. The current manpower shortages within the NHS make it likely that there will be increasing efforts made to accommodate those who do not want to adopt standard job plans. An open attitude to enhancing peoples' working lives is a reputation well worth building as it will attract good staff for future years.

Practical suggestions

- Ask Human Resources to speak to your department about the *Improved Working Lives* initiative in order to familiarise yourself with it.
- Be open to the possibility of alternative working patterns.
- When staff leave the department, find out why - in some cases this may be best done by a sympathetic ear from someone else in the department.
- Act on problems that have caused staff to leave - especially if there is a pattern. This may require altering your own behaviour or challenging that of others.

The Improving Working Lives (IWL) initiative, underpinned by designated standards, commits the NHS to supporting its staff in developing a healthy balance between work and home [1]. It is expected that by April 2003 all NHS employers will have gained accreditation by putting the standards into practice.

Mentoring

Mentoring involves the provision of confidential support to colleagues and can take many forms, both formal and informal. The term normally refers to the relationship between one experienced, established individual (the mentor) with a more junior professional colleague (the mentee) in order to lend support, teaching and guidance.

Some Trusts will have a formal mentoring process whereby individuals can request to be mentored and are therefore paired with a mentor who has agreed to fulfil this role. However, many such relationships also occur naturally within the work environment and can last many years. The relationship is dependent on trust and confidentiality between mentor and mentee. Mentoring can, of course, cross professional and organisational barriers which may bring a new perspective to personal and professional development which is unhindered by internal issues within the Trust.

The process of mentoring can easily appear forced, and previous poor experiences can add to a negative image. But everyone will be able to recall individuals within their own experience and career development who have acted towards him or her as mentors, however one chooses to define mentoring. It may have been an individual who provided the inspiration that led to a particular career path or someone who listened, supported or provided feedback at a difficult time. Each of these interactions gives benefit to the mentee and is the basis for any formal mentoring process.

Many individuals will benefit from a mentor relationship within the workplace. It not only provides support and instruction to the mentee but can also support the professional development of the mentor and enhances good practice within the organisation as a whole. However, for any mentoring scheme to be successful, those entering into it should understand and agree the basic principles underpinning the process. In addition, the process should be supported by the organisation.

Requirements of a mentor

◆ Understanding of and agreement with the purposes of the mentoring scheme.
◆ Relatively experienced.
◆ Respected and holding credibility within the organisation.
◆ Good communication skills.
◆ Knowledgeable about issues relevant to the junior colleague's work.
◆ Able to devote time, interest and energy to the role.
◆ A voluntary participant in the scheme.
◆ Have a commitment to learning and development - and a willingness to learn themselves.
◆ Holding a commitment to quality in their own work and clarity about standards of performance - both clinical and organisational.
◆ Have influence and/or access to influence within the organisation in order to represent the junior colleague.

Practical suggestions

● If you are unsure about the pros and cons of being mentored, find out from Human Resources whether your Trust has a mentoring programme.
● Be willing to offer mentoring to staff within your department, especially new starters.
● Only offer yourself as a mentor to others if you are able to fulfil the requirements of the position.

Appraisal

A fuller description of appraisal techniques is given in the next chapter. However, it is pertinent to stress that appraisal is one way in which it is possible to demonstrate that staff are valued and their contribution is of significance to the functioning of the department. Clinical governance looks towards a process whereby improvements in the quality of healthcare are made across a whole range of activities. Historically, non-clinical aspects of service delivery have received little attention as determinants of good or bad clinical outcomes. That is not to say that hard-working administrative and ancillary staff have not been appreciated but rather that efforts to improve their contribution have been afforded a relatively low priority.

The introduction of appraisal in relation to groups of staff that have not traditionally received much attention can be construed as being threatening or intimidating. However, such anxieties should be readily overcome by an explanation of the rationale of the process. The exchange of ideas and information is likely to be illuminating for managerial and senior clinicians. The actual process which is adopted may vary and evolve over time. If one-to-one appraisal is thought to be too time-consuming or cumbersome, a departmental half-day can be set aside for reviewing the issues faced by different groups of staff. It is reasonable to start each group's session with a short presentation from members of that part of the team; this has the potential to demonstrate the hidden capabilities that exist in any department.

Coping with staff problems

Staff problems come in many different shapes and sizes - conflict, resignation, criminal behaviour, apathy, disciplinary action, suspension, harassment and abuse. Working in the high pressure and emotional environment of a hospital often brings issues like these to the surface, especially when dealing with the many strong and eccentric personalities that inhabit the NHS!

The critical skill for the modern clinician in this aspect of staff management is recognising that there are potential problems brewing and seeking help at an early stage. It is clear that it is not acceptable simply to ignore developing problems that have the potential to lead to patient harm. While we do not inhabit a zero-tolerance world with regard to disruptive or dysfunctional behaviour, the environment is much less tolerant than it once was.

It is now appreciated that it is usually inappropriate to attempt to sort out serious issues of the type mentioned above within a department or unit. The problem or concern should be notified to the appropriate authority (usually the Medical Director, Director of Nursing or Human Resources Director). Early notification of potential difficulties increases the chances of a rapid and effective resolution to the issue; there is a clear move away from a culture of suspension, disciplinary procedures and punishment towards an atmosphere of dispute resolution and problem solving. No one should fail to appreciate that this area is something of a legal minefield and needs to be handled with a high degree of professionalism.

Practical suggestions

- Use your Human Resources department to support and help with conflict issues - don't just try to deal with problems in-house.
- If you are working in a high-risk area (eg. A&E medicine), be trained in handling potentially violent patients.
- If you are in conflict with someone, seek mediation to resolve the issue - don't let it fester.
- Take time out in clinical teams to address tensions lying just under the surface - don't leave them to erupt during the hectic nature of everyday work.
- Is your door open or shut to staff who may have problems to discuss?
- Tackle inappropriate behaviour of colleagues early, before it escalates out of control.

References

1   Human Resources Performance Framework. www.doh.gov.uk/hrstrategy/index.htm.

Further reading

- Working Lives: Programmes for Change. Overview. Department of Health, London. www.doh.gov.uk.
- Good Practice. Workforce and Development. Embodying Leadership in the NHS. Department of Health, London, Oct 2000. www.doh.gov.uk.
- Improving Working Lives Standard. Department of Health, London, 2000. www.doh.gov.uk.
- Supporting doctors and dentists at work: an enquiry into mentoring. Executive Summary, Jan 1998. SCOPME. www.mcgl.dircon.co.uk/scopme/support.htm.
- Improving working lives in the NHS. Department of Health, London, 1999.
- Cook M. New approaches to selecting medical staff. *BMJ* 1998; 316: 7134: 2.
- Rogers J. Recruiting in hard times. *BMJ* 1997; 315: 7122: 2.
- McGuire R. Tips on…conducting work performance appraisals. *BMJ* 2002; 325: S151.
- Grainger C. Mentoring - supporting doctors at work and play. *BMJ* 2002; 324: S203.
- Alred G, Garvey B, Smith R. *The mentoring pocketbook.* Management Pocketbooks, Alresford, 1998.
- King J. Giving feedback. *BMJ* 1999; 318: 7200: 2.
- Sudlow M, Toghill P. How to be interviewed. *BMJ* 1996; 313: 7059: 2.

Chapter 17

Professional development, education and training

If you think education is expensive, try ignorance.
Derek Bok

Doctors, nurses and other healthcare professionals have always been aware of the need to maintain their knowledge base and skills. As the quantity of new data has exploded, the information era has generated huge problems as well as some solutions for the individual who is looking to maintain their professional standards. The introduction of clinical governance into the NHS has changed the landscape from one where high standards were taken for granted in exchange for the privileges of professional status. It is now accepted that external structures and checks are needed in order to guarantee lifelong development; appraisal, assessment and revalidation have been introduced in response to a reduction in confidence in the old values.

One area, which has been clarified in the light of the introduction of clinical governance, is that of the relationship between the individual clinician and their employing organisation. There has been a clear reduction in the degree to which professional development is self-determined. It is now expected that serious consideration will be given to the requirements of the service, as seen by the Trust in question, when the educational and training needs of the practitioner are being examined.

Maintaining clinical expertise

One of the challenges for the clinical governance agenda is to raise the standard of continuing medical education. Many clinicians have an unstructured approach to continuing professional development. We have a tendency to read and attend courses based on what is of interest and what is available at a convenient time - which is often at the end of a busy day. Many will be familiar with the guilt which accompanies the sight of journals, still in their unopened plastic wrappers, gathering dust in a corner. Clinical governance asks for a fresh look at the process of continuing professional development by posing the question: what learning and development is needed to maintain and improve standards of patient care in all the areas in which the practitioner works?

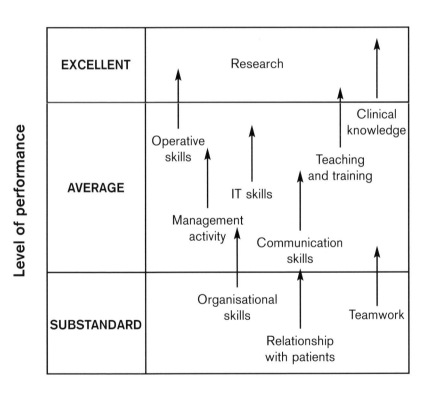

Figure 1. Monitoring individual performance.

The appraisal process should become central to the process of planning continuing professional development. The process should, in theory, identify areas of practice where there might be room for improvement; a plan can then be formulated to overcome these weaknesses. A simple chart (if used honestly!) can provide a useful overview of one's individual performance. Whatever the skills of the individual, the intention should be to always improve one's performance.

Practical suggestions

● Map out the scope of your clinical practice.

● Identify areas that are rusty or underdeveloped - you might need to ask your colleagues (Figure 1).

● Look at available sources of information and training - journal articles, reviews, guidelines, books, courses, meetings and the electronic media.

● Formulate a programme of learning based on the identified needs and the most applicable information resources.

● Keep the plan realistic and achievable.

● Remain focused on the continuing professional development plan - minimise education time spent on work which is not in the targeted areas.

● Keep a note of topics for next year's plan.

By way of illustration, a clinician may decide to meet their background needs by using a review journal and by selecting editorial and review articles in two key specialist journals. They might opt to attend courses on specific topics where their knowledge or skills may need updating. Finally, they might arrange a visit to another unit to augment their knowledge and skills in an area of particular interest that they are planning to incorporate into their practice.

Non-clinical development

The complexity of healthcare provision is such that healthcare management and administration require considerable professional input. There are numerous areas that clinicians may choose to engage with, in addition to their usual clinical duties.

Non-clinical development roles

◆ Departmental administration - the clinical director role.

◆ Trust level management roles - medical director, medical staff committee work, local negotiating committee representation.

◆ Teaching at levels from medical student to post graduate.

◆ Examining at the various levels.

◆ Training committee and Royal College work.

◆ Medico-legal, expert witness work.

◆ Research.

There are incentives within the NHS system that are designed to encourage individuals to take on these additional roles in the form of discretionary points and distinction awards but, for many, the incentive lies either in the interest or status which such activities offer. The difficulty that the non-clinical roles present, lies in their competing for the limited resources of time and energy. The fashion for 'life coaches' has not swept through the healthcare sector but, as generations of clinicians continue to live unbalanced lives, perhaps it should!

Practical suggestions

- Plan non-clinical work. Where do your interests and abilities lie? What are your short, medium and long-term aims?
- Try to timetable this work into specific sessions in your job plan if possible.
- Ensure that adequate support is available for the task - be able to delegate where appropriate.
- Do not take on additional tasks if you cannot accommodate them; learn to say 'no'.
- Non-clinical work requires skill. Get trained in tasks such as chairing a meeting.
- Make room for family life and recreation. Remember that the epitaph "I wish I'd spent more of my life in the office", is rarely used!

Introducing new techniques and procedures

Rapid technological advances have occurred in medical practice in recent years but the introduction of new techniques and procedures has not been entirely straightforward. The introduction of laparoscopy into general surgical practice has been of undoubted benefit but some patients have paid a high price as surgeons move along their learning curves. The problems of introducing complex new paediatric cardiac operations have been extensively documented by the Kennedy report into events in Bristol.

In the field of drug therapy, regulation has been established over a longer period and controls are exerted at national and local levels. Furthermore, independent advice is available from many sources including publications such as the *Drugs and Therapeutic Bulletin* and in the form of guidelines such as those generated by the National Institute of Clinical Excellence (NICE). New surgical procedures are not governed by such stringent statutory controls although those involving implants and devices have some restrictions that are likely to be significantly strengthened as

NICE introduces a registration and guidelines structure. However, it is now clear that the concept of patients being exposed to random learning curves is not acceptable in theory - even though the attainment of that ideal is unlikely to be completely practicable.

Introducing new procedures

For a clinician who is introducing a procedure into their clinical practice the following steps are required:

- Review the evidence of the procedure's efficacy and potential side-effects.
- Ensure that it is applicable to the patient population in question.
- Check that there will be sufficient workload in order to maintain a satisfactory level of expertise.
- Notify and discuss the change of practice and the implementation plan with the clinical director or medical director.
- Plan a training strategy which might entail attendance at a course, visits to other units and the use of mentors visiting the clinician's unit until expertise is established.
- Establish appropriate audit criteria and methodology.

For novel procedures, further considerations apply. If the approach is experimental, ethics committee approval of a formal research protocol will be needed. For procedures that fall in the grey area between the experimental and the established, the NICE *New Interventional Procedures* protocol [1] should be consulted and followed.

Appraisal, assessment and revalidation

Several different forces are driving changes to the way in which professional knowledge and skills are maintained and monitored. On the one hand, healthcare professions are looking at appraisal as a means of structuring and supporting continuing professional development while, on the other hand, assessment and revalidation are being formalised in response to concerns about clinical competence. Several high profile cases of serial incompetence led to the government questioning the ability of the medical profession in general, and the General Medical Council (GMC) in particular, to ensure that doctors maintain high standards throughout their working lives. Revalidation will need to demonstrate that doctors are safe and competent to have a licence to practice. The appraisal and assessment process will look more closely at quality issues and will examine the individual's ability to engage with the clinical governance agenda.

In its purest form appraisal is a process which is supportive and confidential. A fellow professional aids an individual in a process of reflection and consideration; they look at the person's current working circumstances and practice and plan how professional and personal development might be achieved. In contrast, assessment is an exercise in examining and measurement. Assessment aims to clearly define how well an individual is performing in comparison with external standards; it is a fundamentally judgemental process. Revalidation is the procedure that enables a practitioner to remain correctly registered and therefore able to practice. The process of appraisal and revalidation are for the majority of doctors inextricably linked as the annual appraisal process will form a basis on which revalidation decisions will be made [2]. Central to the evidence required for appraisal and revalidation will be the personal portfolio to be developed by each doctor. But, there is a steep learning curve for all doctors in developing these portfolios to support the appraisal process and subsequent revalidation.

In practice, current plans within the medical sphere are biased towards assessment for trainees and appraisal for senior doctors. However, the planned linkage between revalidation and appraisal means that there will undoubtedly be an element of assessment worked into the appraisal mechanism. In the event of a future scandal, the public and media will not be convinced that much has changed if the only effect of new revalidation procedures is to check that a couple of doctors have met once a year for a confidential chat! Trusts will therefore be expected to show that their appraisal systems are effective in forthcoming CHI/CHAI reviews.

It is worth looking at the consultant appraisal process, as this will bear similarities to the way in which the technique is applied to other healthcare groups. The need for consultants to be appraised on an annual basis was announced in an NHS Executive letter in 2000 [3]. Appraisal was characterised as "a professional process of constructive dialogue, in which the doctor being appraised has a formal structured opportunity to reflect on his/her work and to consider how his/her effectiveness might be improved." The aims of the process include the following:

The aims of the appraisal process

◆ To review an individual's work and performance.
◆ To optimise the use of skills and resources.
◆ To agree plans to meet personal and professional development needs.
◆ To identify resource needs in the work environment.
◆ To examine ways in which the individual might contribute to the wider NHS.
◆ To provide documentation which will form the basis for GMC revalidation.

As with so much of the clinical governance agenda, appraisal can only be regarded as a positive development. The devil is in the detail of putting the concept into practice. Particular concerns relate to the extent to which the process is costly in terms of professional time, difficulties with data availability and quality, and the likelihood that sufficient resource will not be available to meet identified personal development needs.

The development of appraisal is following somewhat different courses for the various professional groups. For junior doctors the process often amounts to an exercise in filling in forms. Being signed off as satisfactory from each job is all that is required for entry to college examinations and is not required at all for those not wanting to follow a specific specialist career path. Confusion is seen as a result of a failure always to distinguish the appraisal and assessment functions - are we meant to be supportive or judgemental today?

What goes into an appraisal portfolio?

The contents of a portfolio will vary from individual to individual; the suggested contents of a general practitioner's appraisal documentation are given here as an example. Computerised toolkits are being developed to aid documentation and to help structure the appraisal process. Further information is available at: http://www.appraisaluk.info/

◆ Basic details. GMC number etc.
◆ Audit activity.
◆ Details of significant events.
◆ Prescribing data. Including comparative information.
◆ Learning activities. Covering educational needs, professional development planning and educational activities completed.
◆ Feedback from patients including complaints.
◆ Medical activities and their place in the context of the practice as a whole.
◆ Teaching and training activities.
◆ Probity issues.
◆ Management work.
◆ Research participation.
◆ Personal health issues.

Practical suggestions

- Take control of your own appraisal and make sure that this is performed for you regularly.
- Be prepared for your appraisal - spend time reflecting on what your development needs truly are. Get views from others.
- Develop good skills in giving feedback.
- Make sure you access training for appraisal and use this with your own non-clinical staff
- Whatever level you are at, familiarise yourself with the consultant appraisal forms (Appendix IV).
- Start your professional development portfolio. Collect details of your own work in keeping with the requirements of the appraisal toolkit document - this may mean keeping details of complaints that you were involved in or thank you letters from patients.
- Discuss with other consultant colleagues in your specialty, their approach to developing portfolios.
- Co-ordinate junior audit projects with any relevant national performance indicators for the specialty - this will enable the work to be used for consultant performance assessment.
- Doctors in non-training posts should use the standard Non-Consultant Career Grades (NCCG) appraisal forms.
- Consider carefully whom you would wish to act as your appraiser. Someone from another Trust or organisation may bring fresh ideas and carry more weight with management if they identify particular service needs. However, you would need to clear this with your clinical director.

Teaching and training responsibilities

Teaching and training stand a little to one side from the main thrust of clinical governance but nevertheless cannot be ignored in this context. One of the most powerful instruments of change in healthcare practice has proved to be the alteration in relationship between trainer and trainee. The impact of a new educational agenda was first felt in nursing; student nurses had provided a significant part of the nursing workforce - and at a very competitive price - when Project 2000 curriculum changes took them from the wards into the classroom. For junior doctors the changes have been the result of hours of work legislation as well as alterations in the educational process itself.

The shift from an apprenticeship-based approach to medical and nursing education to a more structured teaching system has not been straightforward. Stresses, which can impact on patient care, remain in the system. Clinical governance indicates that the problems which have arisen must be addressed and resolved. Unfortunately, progress in this area is usually at the cost of reduced patient throughput for any individual clinical team.

For decades, senior NHS staff have accepted the role of trainer as being part of the job. In exchange, the practitioner was provided with a team of willing and loyal juniors who traded their enthusiasm and diligence for a favourable reference. As this system has been dismantled, two pressures have come to bear on the trainers: first, an expectation they will provide more structured training and, second, an increased burden of clinical work as a result of a decreased level of junior support. The need to train ever greater numbers of doctors, nurses and other professionals threatens to put yet more strain on this part of the system and it is conceivable that some senior staff may even opt out of the training role altogether.

What then is the clinical governance impact in this field? Firstly, there is now recognition that training does take time and effort. There is no real option but to make room for the activity by appropriate timetabling. In particular, the role of junior staff has to be considered for individual activities - are they there to be taught (with a time allowance for this) or is their task predominately service-orientated and within their established capabilities?

Changing patterns of service delivery are not always clearly identified. It is important to recognise the impact of changing work patterns and try to prevent problems arising rather than simply reacting to inevitable difficulties. For instance, the introduction of shift systems will impact on continuity of care at a junior doctor level. Protocols for effective handover (so well established in nursing) must be put in place at the inception of any rota changes.

A further area where the introduction of clinical governance has added clarity is that of delegation. Over a period of 20 years, there has been a major change in attitude to delegation. The days of junior surgeons operating out of hours, at, or beyond, their level of experience and competence are gone. However, a healthcare professional must have experience of working without continuous supervision if they are to take on the role of an independent practitioner on completion of training. This is therefore an area where careful judgements have to be made. Delegation of clinical tasks must be undertaken with the patient's welfare as the primary, but not sole, concern. There should be good grounds for thinking that the trainee can competently complete the task and, in addition, the trainee must be aware of their responsibility to summon help if difficulties arise. Finally, that assistance must be readily accessible and freely given.

Practical suggestions

- Use a departmental meeting to review and evaluate how junior members of the team are being trained.
- Try to timetable formal teaching into your job plan.
- Go on a 'training the trainer' course - make sure that you are up to speed with training techniques.
- Be aware that overbooked clinical sessions are bad for patients and bad for training.
- Do not forget to delegate but delegate thoughtfully.
- Look to other specialties for examples of good practice.

References

1   NICE - New Interventional Procedures. www.nice.org.uk/catlist.asp?c=29553.
2   A Licence to Practice and Revalidation. GMC, London, 2003.
3   Consultants contract: annual appraisal for consultants. Advance Letter (MD) 6/2000. www.doh.gov.uk/consultantcontract.htm.

Further reading

*   A strategy for continuing education and professional development for hospital doctors and dentists. A SCOPME Report 1999. www.mcgl.dircon.co.uk/scopme/index.htm.
*   Learning from Bristol: The DH Response to the Report of the Public Inquiry into children's heart surgery at the Bristol Royal Infirmary 1984-1995. Annex A. Recommendations and Responses. www.doh.gov.uk.
*   Learning from Bristol: The DH Response to the Report of the Public Inquiry into children's heart surgery at the Bristol Royal Infirmary 1984-1995, Chapter 7. The Regulation and Education of Health Care Professionals. www.doh.gov.uk.
*   Peyton JWR. Appraisal and assessment in surgical practice. *Ann R Coll Surg Engl* (Suppl) 2002; 84: 350-351.
*   Working Together - Learning Together: a framework for lifelong learning for the NHS. Department of Health, London, Nov 2001. www.doh.gov.uk.
*   McGuire R. Tips on...conducting work performance appraisals. *BMJ* 2002; 325: S151.
*   King J. Giving feedback. *BMJ* 1999; 318: 7200-2.
*   General Medical Council. Proposals for revalidation. GMC, London, 2000.
*   Du Boulay C. Revalidation for doctors in the United Kingdom: the end or the beginning? *BMJ* 2000; 320: 1490.
*   King J. 360° appraisal. *BMJ* 2002; 324: S195.
*   British Association of Medical Managers. Appraisal In Action. British Association of Medical Managers, 1999.
*   Department of Health. Postgraduate Medical Education and Training: The Medical Education Standards Board. The Stationery Office, London, 2001.

Chapter 18

Consultation and patient involvement

*There would never be any public agreement
among doctors if they did not agree to agree on the main point
of the doctor being always in the right.*
George Bernard Shaw

Quality from the patient perspective

Quality in healthcare has two distinct dimensions. Firstly, it can be determined as excellence in diagnostic, therapeutic, clinical management techniques and improved health outcomes. It is quality in these terms that most healthcare professionals would aspire to and be most concerned with. The second dimension concerns the quality of the patient's experience of care. This aspect has come to the fore in recent years and can only be determined by patients themselves as receivers of the care provided.

It was clear from the earliest guidance on clinical governance, that patient experience would be a key performance indicator within the overall framework for building increased quality into the NHS. More generally, there was awareness that re-building public confidence in the NHS was a fundamental cornerstone of the government's policy for a modernised NHS. This would include making the service more accountable to patients and being shaped by their views.

This chapter focuses on one particular aspect of patient involvement - that of the drive for NHS organisations to engage with patients and the public in its wider decision-making. We have already looked at the changed nature of the individual doctor-patient relationship in chapters 12 and 13.

Getting patients involved

Governments have been pushing for increased patient involvement in both planning and providing NHS services for many years. Until recently, local NHS organisations have been essentially left to their own devices to take this forward. As a result there have been many haphazard and varied attempts at gaining patient views. A wealth of non-standardised information has been produced from local patient surveys, interviews and diaries and for what gain? Undoubtedly there have been localised successful examples of where patient feedback has achieved change. But this has not been seen universally.

Effective patient representation has always been an elusive goal for all NHS organisations. Many models and approaches have been tried across different NHS organisations. Attempts to engage patient interest through focus groups would often last only through the planning stages of any hospital development, without any hope of sustaining user involvement thereafter. Patient Participation Groups, a model developed in primary care, seemed to hold promise but inevitably was too reliant on the continued involvement of certain individuals - usually those who championed the role of the group from the outset.

The impact of this relatively *ad hoc* approach to patient involvement across the NHS was felt most by those who represented the public/patient's perspective on various committees in local NHS organisations. These lay positions often became isolated ways of attempting to show patient and public involvement. Such positions, in the absence of a more structured and systematic process readily become viewed as tokenistic.

All these experiences, driven by an initial measure of scepticism, may have generated disillusionment amongst clinicians and managers regarding the value of patient feedback as a driver of change in healthcare provision.

A new national approach

The modernisation drive is looking towards a change in the current levels of patient involvement in healthcare delivery, planning and policy.

Patients are now recognised as experts in their own right especially in the management of chronic disease [1]. Education and training now aims to bring a non-paternalistic atmosphere to the patient consultation with shared decision-making at the fore.

Radical and complex changes to formal patient and public involvement structures at national, regional and local level are also proposed to define a model that is expected to produce a 'step change' in the levels of meaningful involvement in the NHS. The ground is being cleared by the abolition of local Community Health Councils (CHCs) as the statutory public/patient representative bodies; this has been an immediately controversial aspect of the changes.

Whether these plans achieve the holy grail of true patient/public involvement remains to be seen. Indeed, it is still not clear to many healthcare professionals what is meant by successful patient involvement. How will we know that we have reached this elusive goal? The plans for better public/patient involvement in the new NHS centre are complex and have been criticised by many for this very reason. Will the average person know how their voice can be heard through the complex infrastructure being proposed?

Figure 1 shows how these functions inter-relate at a local level.

Improving patient/public involvement

The approach relies on four main elements to be in place by April 2003.

◆ Reliable information on patient experience.
◆ Resolving patient concerns and supporting complaints.
◆ Establishing strong patient representation.
◆ Developing explicit local public scrutiny.

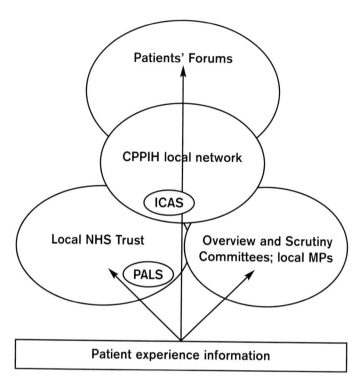

ICAS: Independent Complaints Advocacy Service
PALS: Patient Advice and Liaison Service
CPPIH: Commission for Patient and Public Involvement in Health

Figure 1. Arrangements for patient and public involvement at a local level.
(© *Crown Copyright. Involving Patients and the Public in Healthcare: Response to the Listening Exercise. Department of Health Publications, June 2001).*

Patient experience

For the first time there will be national, co-ordinated surveys of patient experience across primary and secondary care to replace the previous *ad hoc* approach of local patient surveys, interviews and diaries. The NHS Plan requires all NHS and Primary Care Trusts to carry out these local surveys to ask both patients and carers for their views on NHS services. This information is to be gathered in a structured and standardised way

181

18 Consultation and patient involvement

and will feed directly into star ratings for Acute and Primary Care Trusts. The presence of such information is aimed at forcing the patient experience to the top of the priority pile.

Patient feedback surveys

For the first year, hospital Trusts are expected to carry out a patient feedback survey meeting the following requirements:

◆ A postal questionnaire survey.

◆ The questionnaire must be sent to 850 adult inpatients recently discharged from the Trust (excluding maternity and psychiatry patients).

◆ The questionnaire must include 58 core questions which cover the following topics [2]:

  ➤ Admission to hospital.

  ➤ The hospital and ward.

  ➤ Nurses and doctors.

  ➤ Patient care and treatment.

  ➤ Pain.

  ➤ Discharge procedures.

  ➤ Overall evaluation.

  ➤ Patient background and health status.

◆ The response rate must be at least 60% i.e. there must be 500 returned (and valid) questionnaires.

◆ The data must be submitted on time to a central data processing unit.

It is important that local departments and individual clinicians are made aware of the results of their Trust's survey particularly for questions regarding staff attitudes and information given to patients. It is possible in the future that individual Trusts could extend their survey numbers on core questions to target patients discharged from specific departments.

> ### Practical suggestions
>
> - Make sure that your department is aware of the results of your Trust survey.
> - Consider seriously what you can learn from the results, especially if patients have reported problems with staff attitudes or information.
> - Proactively request that further questions and sub-analysis be included by your Trust in future years to give relevant comparisons across departments within the Trust. There is a large bank of extra questions on the same website as the basic 58 question survey.
> - Use the same questionnaire bank within your department to highlight any departmental problem areas - this could perhaps be done as a junior audit project with the Trust results as the set standard against which you compare your department.

Patient concerns and complaints

Every NHS and Primary Care Trust has set up a Patient Advice and Liaison Service (PALS) designed to provide on the spot help for patients within Trusts.

The PALS is not a complaints service. The current complaints procedures for NHS organisations will still exist but has just been reviewed [3]. The current procedure is summarised on page 184 [4]:

Community Health Councils have played an important advocacy role for patients during the complaints process. Now they are to be abolished, patients will be able to access independent advocacy support through a new service, the Independent Complaints Advocacy Services (ICAS). This is to be commissioned through a new national body called the Commission for Patient and Public Involvement in Health (CPPIH). Local

The role of PALS

◆ Providing information to patients, carers and families about health and health services locally.
◆ Putting patients in contact with relevant voluntary organisations and support groups.
◆ Resolving problems and concerns quickly where possible, before they become more serious.
◆ Informing people of the NHS complaints procedure, and putting them in touch with specialist, independent advocacy services when they wish to complain formally.
◆ Acting as an early warning system for Trusts and their Patients' Forums (see below) by monitoring problems in services and staff training.
◆ Submitting anonymised reports for action by Trusts and Patients' Forums.
◆ Working in a network with other PALS in their area to ensure patients' concerns are handled properly when their care has crossed different parts of the service.

providers will be identified to undertake this complaints advocacy work e.g. Citizen's Advice Bureaux.

Patient representation

The most radical change proposed for the modernised NHS is the establishment of Patients' Forums for each NHS and Primary Care Trust. These will be independent statutory bodies. A member of the Patients' Forum will be selected to be a non-executive director of the relevant NHS Trust.

The NHS complaints procedure

◆ Patient complains either within six months of the event, or within six months of realising that there may be grounds for complaint.

◆ Local efforts to deal with the matter at source by those involved eg. doctors, nurses.

◆ If the complaint cannot be immediately resolved the complainant is encouraged to put the complaint in writing.

◆ Complaint received by the designated Complaints Manager within the Trust.

◆ Complaint is responded to in writing within the designated time.

◆ If a complaint cannot satisfactorily be answered in writing there are various options open to Trusts:

➤ Local resolution by further discussion.

➤ Lay conciliation.

➤ An Independent Review Panel - the decision to proceed to this rests with the Complaints Convenor, a non-executive director of the Trust Board, together with a lay chairperson appointed by the NHS Executive *.

◆ If a complainant remains dissatisfied with the outcome of a review panel, or in cases where a review panel was refused, they have the option to refer their complaint to the Ombudsman.

---

* The recent review of the NHS complaints system has proposed that Independent Review Panels are to be run in future by the Commission for Healthcare Audit and Inspection (CHAI).

The role of the Patients' Forum

◆ Representing the views of local communities to Trusts, about the quality and configuration of health services by actively engaging in the community to find out what patients, carers and families think.
◆ Monitoring service delivery from the patient's perspective including an active inspection role.
◆ Producing an annual report of its work and making its findings and reports available not only to Trusts, but also bodies such as the local Overview and Scrutiny Committees (see below), local MPs, and the relevant Strategic Health Authority.
◆ Monitoring the quality of the Trust's PALS.

Practical suggestions

● Invite your general manager, or a representative, to run through your departmental complaints with the department once a month; don't deal with them purely at a senior level.
● Involve all within the department in playing a role in reducing justified patient complaints.
● Invite the complaints manager to give training in dealing with complaints.
● Ask the PALS officer to talk to your department about their work and any issues that have arisen from their contacts with patients concerning the work of your department.
● It is worth remembering that the majority of complaints come from people because they care about the NHS.

Public scrutiny

With the abolition of the CHCs there is a need to ensure there is a broad scrutiny role of the work of the NHS locally. This will be achieved by the establishment of Overview and Scrutiny Committees (OSCs) within Local Authorities comprising local councillors as democratically elected representatives of the local population.

Their role will be to scrutinise and challenge, where appropriate, local NHS provision as part of the wider role for all Local Authorities to promote well-being and health improvement and reduce health inequalities for their area and its inhabitants. NHS managers will likely find this a challenging process, as OSCs will want to call them to account for their actions and decisions.

Part of the role will also be to have formal powers to refer significant public concerns over major health service changes (or poorly conducted consultations) to the Secretary of State for Health; this represents continuation of the arrangement whereby CHCs could refer controversial planning issues directly to the minister, such as hospital closures.

What does all this mean to clinicians?

Many clinicians will find it difficult not to view this aspect of clinical governance in a particularly sceptical light; there are real practical difficulties in involving lay individuals in the process of making important, complex and technical decisions. The issue of patient involvement is often accompanied by a strong whiff of political correctness. The concept seems to be intuitively right and proper but somehow fails to solidify into a practical, substantial reality. Even if the topic is approached with an open mind, the question remains to be answered as to whether this is an area that individual units and departments can usefully engage with.

So we have all these new formal patient and public involvement structures. However, it is still difficult for individual clinicians and their teams to access information from patients and to put such data to good effect - in terms of service improvement. Trusts will need to filter patient information down through the system effectively if the resource is going to be put to best use.

However, patient and user feedback from formal structured sources like the Trust's annual patient survey or PALS will not always tell clinicians everything they need to know. At times it will be necessary and appropriate to gain more detailed information about individual services or members of staff.

To seek information independently of the formalised structures requires careful consideration and discussion if time and effort is not to be wasted. It is all too easy to rush out doing interviews and hand out questionnaires without establishing first the ways such information can and cannot be utilised and secondly to make sure the information isn't already available. A case for definitely needing to work smarter! Once again, experience with conducting research is relevant; issues of questionnaire validation and analysis are familiar to those who have collected data regarding patients' symptoms and their response to therapeutic interventions.

If patient consultation is to be carried out effectively there must be both a tried and tested method for data collection as well as a robust plan for how the data will effect change. The responsibility for this must lie at the feet of the individuals carrying out the data collection. If it does not, then the exercise remains one of potentially meaningless observation.

There are a host of mechanisms for seeking patients' views, each with their own pros and cons. Table 1 summarises some of the possibilities open to us [5].

Table 1. The possibilities for seeking patients' views.

	Pros	Cons
Casual observations	No cost	Observer may misinterpret events Observations may not be representative of all patients
Systematic observation	Low cost Unobtrusive Can be done quickly	Observers may misinterpret events Observations may not be representative
In-depth interviews and discovery interviews	Provide patients' perspective on complex issues Use patients' own words First-hand accounts can provide persuasive results Flexible	Labour intensive Subject to interviewer bias Expensive Do not produce quantifiable data
Patient diaries	Patients can describe experiences in their own words Patients can focus on the issues that are important to them Immediate recording of events can improve accuracy of patient reports	Do not produce quantifiable data Data analysis is labour intensive Analysis and interpretation is subject to researcher bias
Focus groups	Provide patients' perspective of complex issues Allow exploration of issues Flexible Take advantage of synergy among patients Can provide insight into why opinions are held Can help reveal degree or lack of consensus Appropriate for populations with low levels of literacy	Results may not be generalisable Participants with strong views can bias the results Do not produce quantifiable data
Questionnaire surveys	Can be more representative (sample sizes are often larger) Questions can be standardised Easy to replicate and compare Administration method can be adapted to purpose and population	Limited scope for exploring complex issues Assume knowledge and understanding of patients' problems Some populations may be difficult to reach

---

Practical suggestions

- Plan how you will effect change as a result of potentially unfavourable patient views.
- Foster a culture where it is seen as OK for patients to raise concerns or suggest changes.
- Don't be tempted to ask patients about everything, as there will be many elements of care that you cannot change.
- Use standardised questionnaires unless you have a lot of experience of writing questionnaires.
- If you need to write your own questionnaire, you must pilot it and assess the results - there are bound to be questions that are unclear, could have multiple answers and thus make future analysis difficult.
- Make sure you are asking a representative sample of patients - there are numerous statistics books and websites that will give you an introduction into sampling techniques. But, the comments of an individual can still be powerful in their own right.
- Don't attempt to gather informal communication from more than one source, as it will be impossible within the normal working environment of the NHS.
- Don't dismiss informal communication about departmental performance. It is still useful in its own respect.
- Secretaries can collect data about informal communication from discussions with patients on the office phone, outpatient receptionist from face-to-face discussions with patients, nurses at the point of patient discharge.

(Table 1 on facing page. © Crown Copyright. Listening To Your Patients. NHS Trust-based Patient Surveys: Inpatients - acute hospitals. Department of Health Publications, 2002. Reproduced with the kind permission of the Advice Centre for the NHS Patient Survey Programme).

References

1   Department of Health. The Expert Patient: A new approach to chronic disease management in the 21st century. The Stationery Office, London, 2001. www.doh.gov.uk/cmo/ep-report.pdf.

2   www.pickereurope.org/nhstrustsurveys.

3   NHS Complaints Reform - Making things right. Department of Health Publications, March 2003.

4   Campbell B, Callum K, Peacock NA. *Operating Within The Law. A practical guide for surgeons and lawyers.* tfm Publishing Ltd, Shrewsbury, 2001.

5   Listening To Your Patients. NHS Trust-based Patient Surveys: Inpatients - acute hospitals. Department of Health Publications, 2002. www.doh.gov.uk/acutesurvey.

Further reading

•   Involving Patients and the Public in Healthcare: Response to the Listening Exercise. Department of Health Publications, June 2001. www.doh.gov.uk/involvingpatients.

•   Complaints Procedures for the Department of Health, 2000. www.doh.gov.uk/complaints/index.htm.

•   Patient Experience. *Clinical Governance Bulletin* July 2000; Vol 1(1).

•   Crawford MJ, Rutter D, Manley C, Weaver T, Bhui K, Fulop N, *et al.* Systematic review of involving patients in the planning and development of healthcare. *BMJ* 2002; 325: 1263-1265.

•   Secretary of State for Health. The new NHS, modern, dependable. The Stationery Office, London, 1997(Cm 3807).

•   Department of Health. The NHS plan: a plan for investment, a plan for reform. The Stationery Office, Norwich, 2000.

•   NHS Executive. Patient and public involvement in the new NHS. Department of Health, Leeds, 1999.

Authors' endnote

Final thoughts

In the preface the authors described this book as an exploration of clinical governance five years on after its introduction. These final paragraphs contain some of the observations which we have made during our journey (some readers may consider 'ramble' to be a more apt description) through this changing landscape.

Firstly, the introduction of clinical governance does seem to represent a truly revolutionary process; the structures and concepts are not all new but there can be no doubt that the face of medical practice is being changed in a radical manner. The belief that self-imposed professional standards are sufficient to protect healthcare quality has lost its credibility with the public, the media and politicians. But the process is not just about controlling the various groups of medical professionals; it is a genuine and forceful attempt to improve quality in the NHS.

A massive administrative effort, and significant financial backing, has supported the launch of clinical governance. The sheer volume of material, which has been produced by the Department of Health and others, is extraordinary - with much of it being praiseworthy. Perhaps there should be no surprise that it is difficult to disagree with much of the material that has been produced; after all, we should all be interested in providing high quality healthcare. The effort that has been made should therefore be acknowledged as an important and major contribution.

The context in which clinical governance has been developed as a concept leads, inevitably, to the feeling that it is being imposed and represents an additional burden to hard-pressed clinicians and managers. To some extent this view is correct but it is vital that those of us on the 'shop floor' realise that clinical governance invests considerable power in the individual clinician. Clinical governance is the counter-balance to the pressures that have driven healthcare for too long, namely cost-containment and performance targets.

There is substantial room for optimism in view of the fact that the need to increase the quality of healthcare delivery has been so vigorously considered. However, it is difficult not to be apprehensive about the future. The political status of the NHS leaves it open to a process of continued tinkering and adjustment as the history of repeated reorganisation demonstrates. Those in power now need to have the courage to let the recent NHS upheavals settle by establishing a period of evolution. Furthermore, the workforce needs to see evidence that realism and practicality are tempering the reforming zeal; quality improvement does not always consume time and resources but often it does. Therefore, it must be acknowledged that the NHS is currently awash with insoluble equations involving performance targets, quality improvements and limited financial and manpower resources; change must be prioritised and timetabled into a realistic and attainable programme which integrates the need to treat large numbers of patients expeditiously with the requirement also to treat them well.

And, finally…. an admission. We have tried to point towards a practical approach to clinical governance with advice and suggestions. It would seem dishonest not to admit that in many areas we continue to fail to put our own preaching into practice. In mitigation we would wish to point out that at least we now recognise where we are failing to live up to the expectations of those who have been directing the development of clinical governance.

Appendix I

Key websites

The Department of Health	http://www.doh.gov.uk
National Institute of Clinical Excellence	http://www.nice.org.uk
National Health Service	http://www.nhs.uk
Commission for Health Improvement	http://www.chi.nhs.uk
National Patient Safety Agency	http://www.npsa.nhs.uk
National Electronic Library for Health	http://www.nelh.nhs.uk
The Cochrane Library	http://www.cochrane.org
Centre for Evidence Based Medicine	http://www.cebm.net
National Guideline Clearinghouse	http://www.guideline.gov
Bandolier	http://www.jr2.ox.ac.uk/bandolier

Royal Society of Medicine Publishing supplying: *On-line journals*
Clinical Governance Bulletin
Clinical Risk
Effective Health Care
& others at http://www.rsm.ac.uk

BMJ Publishing Group supplying: *On-line journals*
Evidence Based Products
Clinical Evidence
CME/CPD at http://www.bmjpg.com

The Bristol Inquiry	http://www.bristol-inquiry.org.uk
Response to Bristol	http://www.doh.gov.uk/bristolinquiryresponse

Appendix II
Key NHS agencies

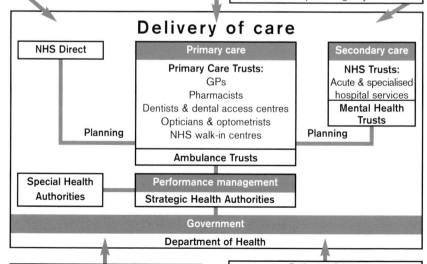

System redesign
- Modernisation Agency
  - Clinical Governance Support Team
  - National Leadership Centres
  - National Primary and Care Trust Development Programme
- NHS Information Authority
  - National Electronic Library for Health

Auditing, assessing & monitoring
- National Clinical Assessment Authority
- Commission for Health Improvement
- National Care Standards Commission
- Audit Commission
- National Audit Office
- Health Ombudsman
- Professional Regulatory Bodies

Standard setting and guidelines
- National Institute for Clinical Excellence
  - National Prescribing Centre
  - National Collaborating Centres
  - Confidential Enquiry Bodies
  - National Co-ordinating Centre for Health Technology Assessment
- Royal Colleges
- Professional Regulatory Bodies
- Health Development Agency

Delivery of care

NHS Direct

Primary care

Primary Care Trusts:
GPs
Pharmacists
Dentists & dental access centres
Opticians & optometrists
NHS walk-in centres

Secondary care

NHS Trusts:
Acute & specialised hospital services

Mental Health Trusts

Planning

Planning

Ambulance Trusts

Special Health Authorities

Performance management

Strategic Health Authorities

Government

Department of Health

Patient involvement
- Commission for Patient and Public Involvement in Healthcare

Patient safety
- National Patient Safety Agency
- Medicines and Healthcare products Regulatory Agency

Appendix III
Audit decision tool

Project Initiation Form - Question/Answer Guide

1) Topic: **What do you want to investigate?**

Examples:		
A particular intervention	How care is documented	Levels of knowledge

2) Background: **Why do you want to investigate?**

Examples:
Critical/clinical incident data   Outcomes   Uncertainty over best practice
Complaints (formal)   Suspected variation in practice
Published information (new guidelines, national guidance)

3) What are the 'drivers' for this work? eg. internal, external

Examples:

Internal drivers   the 'team'

External drivers   Divisional/directorate management,
            Trust initiative, Royal Colleges,
            Professional bodies, Audit Commission

4) Standards: **What is current best practice?**

Examples:
Literature search   National guidance (NICE)   In house guidelines
Benchmarks   National Service Frameworks
(national, local, regional)

5) **What is/are the best source(s) of information to measure your current practice?**

> **Examples:**
> Case notes/nursing records   Database   Staff questionnaire
> Focus groups   Critical/clinical incident data
> Complaints (formal)   Outcome data

6) **Predicted implications for change/improvement in practice: How might change be initiated?**

> **Examples:**
> Education/training   Dissemination   Information/publicity

How will you know if improvement has occurred?

> Look back at original data sources, can these be revisited?
> eg. outcomes, incidents, documentation

7) **Participation, sponsorship and support: Who needs to be involved, and at what level?**

> **Examples:**
> Multi-disciplinary team   Community/GP   PCT
> Management   Risk management   Patients/carers

> **Examples:**
> Full active participation   Responsible/lead   Informed of progress
> Consulted

8) **The audit cycle: How can the team ensure that best practice and the recommendations and action points from this audit are carried out and maintained?**

> **Examples:**
> Agree review programme (eg. periodic updating of evidence base)
> Ongoing monitoring - electronic database, regular documentation review
> Establishment of an integrated care pathway
> Participation in national/local benchmarking programme
> **Do you have the team 'on board' for your audit project?**

Reproduced with the kind permission of G Richardson, Pinderfields General Hospital, The Mid Yorkshire Hospitals NHS Trust.

Appendix IV
Consultant appraisal forms

Every consultant being appraised has been advised to prepare an appraisal folder. This is a systematically recorded set of documents which will help inform the appraisal process. National Guidance on this process has been given to encourage consistency between all consultants year on year.

Forms 1-4 are forwarded to the Chief Executive as a summary of the appraisal outcome and will also form the basis of the revalidation process. The following summarises these forms which are available at: www.doh.gov.uk/nhsexec/consultantappraisal.

FORM 1 - Background details

The aim of this section is to provide:

● basic background personal information;
● brief details of career and professional status;
● any other personal details describing current practice eg. membership of medical and specialist societies.

FORM 2 - Details of current medical activities

The aim of this section is to provide an opportunity to describe post(s) in the NHS, in other public sector bodies, or in the private sector, including titles and grades of any posts currently held, or held in the past year.

It can include comments on the practice environment, including:

- factors believed to affect the provision of good healthcare, including resources available;
- action taken to address any obstacles to the provision of good healthcare.

FORM 3 - Record of reference documentation supporting the appraisal and report on development action in the past year

The aim of this section is to record the background evidence and information that will help to inform appraisal discussions. This should include all fields of practice within the NHS including management, research responsibilities and work in more than one specialty. The headings of *Good Medical Practice* provide the framework for the collection of information and evidence for appraisal discussion.

1. Good medical care
2. Maintaining good medical practice (i.e. record of CPD/CME activities undertaken since the last appraisal).
3. Working relationships with colleagues
4. Relations with patients
5. Teaching and training
6. Probity
7. Health

A summary of progress on the Personal Development Plan agreed at the last appraisal (or at any interim meeting) is included in this section.

FORM 4 - Summary of appraisal discussion with agreed action and personal development plan

The aim of this section is to provide an agreed summary of the appraisal discussion based on the documents listed in Form 3 and a description of the action agreed in the course of the appraisal, including those forming the personal development plan.

This form is completed by the appraiser and agreed by the appraisee. Under each heading the appraiser explains which of the documents listed in Form 3 informed this part of the discussion, the conclusion reached and say what if any action has been agreed.

In the Personal Development Plan part of this section the appraiser and appraisee identify key development objectives for the year ahead relating to the appraisee's personal and/or professional development. This will include action identified in the summary above but may also include other development activity, for example, where this arises as part of discussions on objectives and job planning. Timescales will be agreed for the various aspects of the Personal Development Plan.

FORM 5 - Personal and organisational effectiveness

The aim of this section is to describe individual effectiveness on a personal level and within the NHS organisation with a view to informing job plan review. The appraiser should also prepare a workload summary with the appraisee.

FORM 6 - Detailed confidential account of appraisal interview

This voluntary section is to provide an opportunity to record a fuller, more detailed account of the appraisal discussion than that recorded on Form 4 and which both parties feel may inform or help the next appraisal round. It is confidential (unlike Form 4 which is copied to the Chief Executive).